PERSUADING PEOPLE TO HAVE SAFER SEX

Applications of Social Science to the AIDS Crisis

LEA's Communication Series
Jennings Bryant/Dolf Zillmann, General Editors

Selected titles in Applied Communication (Teresa L. Thompson, Advisory Editor) include:

Beck/Ragan/du Pre • Partnership for Health: Building Relationships Between Women and Health Caregivers

Elwood • Power in the Blood: A Handbook on AIDS, Politics, and Communication, Second Edition

Nussbaum/Pecchioni/Robinson/Thompson • Communication and Aging, Second Edition

Ray • Communication and Disenfranchisement: Social Health Issues and Implications

Street/Gold/Manning • Health Promotion and Interactive Technology: Theoretical Applications and Future Directions

Whaley • Explaining Illness: Research, Theory, and Strategy

For a complete list of titles in LEA's Communication Series, please contact Lawrence Erlbaum Associates, Publishers

PERSUADING PEOPLE
TO HAVE
SAFER SEX

Applications of Social Science
to the AIDS Crisis

RICHARD M. PERLOFF
Cleveland State University

 LAWRENCE ERLBAUM ASSOCIATES, PUBLISHERS
2001   Mahwah, New Jersey   London

Lawrence Erlbaum Associates, Inc., Publishers
10 Industrial Avenue
Mahwah, NJ 07430

Cover design by Kathryn Houghtaling Lacey

Library of Congress Cataloging-in-Publication Data

Perloff, Richard M.
   Persuading people to have safer sex : applications of social science to the AIDS crisis /
Richard M. Perloff.
      p.   cm.
   Includes bibliographical references and indexes.
   ISBN 0–8058–3380–3 (cloth) — ISBN 0–8058–3381–1 (pbk.)
      1. Safe sex in AIDS prevention. 2. AIDS (Disease)–Prevention–Social aspects.
   3. Health behavior. 4. Persuasion (Psychology)   I. Title.
   RA644.A25 P43 2000
   362.1'969792—dc21   00–058759

Books published by Lawrence Erlbaum Associates are printed on acid-free paper,
and their bindings are chosen for strength and durability.

Printed in the United States of America

10 9 8 7 6 5 4 3 2 1

Contents

Preface   vii

1   Introduction   1

2   Cognitive Foundations of AIDS Prevention Behavior   15

3   Social Psychological and Communication Perspectives on Unsafe Sex   32

4   Culture, Poverty, and AIDS   49

5   Applying Persuasion Theories to AIDS Prevention   68

6   AIDS Prevention Campaigns   94

7   AIDS Stigma and Persuasion   124

References   135

Author Index   151

Subject Index   157

Preface

There is something tragic, horrifying, and (truth be told) deeply engrossing about human misfortune. Scholars have speculated that humans are fascinated by tragedy because it helps us deal with our own vulnerabilities and mortality (Goldenberg et al., 1999). We are at once intrigued, moved, and deeply saddened by tragic events, particularly those that happen suddenly, without apparent cause, and that afflict good people. Such is the case with AIDS.

AIDS occurred during a time when scientists thought they had won the battle against infectious disease—when we thought epidemics were events of the past. Epidemics were things that affected other people from earlier, less intelligent eras—not us, not our people, not today. Then AIDS struck and shattered these illusions. AIDS also reminded us that when it comes to death and disease we are not the rational, mature people we like to think we are. Instead, as human beings, we fall prey to worry, denial, prejudice, and in some cases hateful reactions toward individuals who have contracted the AIDS virus.

Life being complex, HIV/AIDS has also brought out the best in people. Individuals who have contracted the virus have shown courage—even nobility—in coping with disease. Family members have displayed unceasing love and dedication. At the same time, counselors, social scientists, and communication practitioners have shown compassion and wisdom in devising interventions to help people protect themselves against HIV infection.

So the story of AIDS is not a simple one. Nor is it one that is always marked by defeatism and depression. But it is a uniquely human story—one that fundamentally requires us to apply the powers of the mind to help master irrational fears, seemingly uncontrollable emotions, and sexual habits of the heart. These issues intrigued me as a persuasion scholar, and as someone who has long been interested in how people reason when they are experiencing strong emotions and how communications can influence people's thoughts and deep-seated feelings.

AIDS prevention appealed to me because it connected with these intellectual interests and offered me an opportunity to write an integrative book on a topic that matters a great deal. I became acquainted with AIDS preventive communication in the late 1980s when I helped develop a campaign directed at injecting drug users and their sex partners. I maintained my interest and chose to broaden it by delving into the voluminous literature on AIDS, social psychology, and communication.

Like many books, this one tries to reach several audiences. I hope that scholars and educated people who come across it gain insight into why safer sex communication often fails, how we can better persuade people to protect themselves from HIV infection, and how different academic literatures can be synthesized to enhance understanding of a complex phenomenon.

I also direct this book at students—undergraduate and graduate students enrolled in social science courses that apply theory to health or AIDS prevention. Students: I recognize you may approach this topic with a negative bias, having been bombarded by AIDS and safe sex in high school or before. I can understand your fatigue. But I ask that you try to look at the problem a little differently—not as a kid trying to navigate your way through treacherous sexual waters, but as a grownup and budding intellectual seeking insight into the psychology of AIDS prevention. I hope you learn more about the reasons people do not always take precautions against HIV infection, why they do and don't practice safer sex, social and cultural barriers to HIV prevention, and how we can use theory and research to devise more effective health communication campaigns. Perhaps along the way you will learn more about your own feelings toward safer sex, AIDS, and people who have contracted HIV.

In writing this book, I have tried to be thorough. I have also tried not to shy away from controversies, ethical dilemmas, and even graphic descriptions of sexual activity. Some of you may be put off initially by such discussions, but as you read I think you will appreciate the need to openly discuss why some people choose unsafe sex.

ACKNOWLEDGMENTS

I am grateful to many people for their kindness and help. I appreciate the efforts of the Cleveland State University Interlibrary Loan staff and those at the CSU Library (particularly Margaret G. Fox, Patrice Johnson, Marsha Davis-Murphy, Johnnie Spates, and Dominic Tortelli). You made sure I received needed books and articles on AIDS.

I thank colleagues who kindly read or commented on my chapters: Icek Ajzen, Hortensia Amaro, Jim Dearing, William Fisher, Jeffrey Kelly, Edward Maibach, Suzanne Thompson, Diana Stover Tillinghast, Gina Wingood, and Kim Witte.

Sharon J. Muskin is due thanks for word-processing numerous computer disks, drafts, and editing changes with patience, skill, and considerable precision.

I also thank Jennings Bryant for his encouragement and Linda Bathgate, my editor at Lawrence Erlbaum Associates, for standing by me on the AIDS book, offering prompt and reinforcing comments, and making me feel good about my work on the project.

I thank my father-in-law, Jerry Krevans, and mother-in-law, Selma Krevans, for their warm comments and lively conversations.

I am thankful to my dad, Robert Perloff, and mom, Evelyn Perloff, for their kind, wonderful support and efforts to keep me abreast of AIDS articles they came across. My dad's regular sending of papers was enough to fill a file folder.

Finally, I thank my family. My son, Michael, was great, showing more interest in this esoteric project than any 10-year-old I know, interspersing conversations with impressive comments about his own interest of the time: James Bond, 007. My 3-year-old daughter, Catherine—always enthusiastic, effervescent, and positive—made me laugh and appreciate life. My wife, Julie, was wonderful in offering her ear to many conversations about AIDS, ethics, and research. I appreciate her love and wise counsel.

One other group of individuals deserves mention—those who have suffered valiantly with AIDS, and the many counselors, advocates, and committed scientists who work to help people cope with HIV infection and endeavor to persuade others to stay AIDS-free. I have read and thought extensively about your activities and admire your courage. This book is dedicated to you.

—*Richard M. Perloff*

CHAPTER ONE

Introduction

When someone mentions AIDS, what comes to mind? A global epidemic? A terrible human tragedy? Unsafe, promiscuous sex? A topic you'd rather not think of?

AIDS is all these things to people. "AIDS," notes George Whitmore (1988), "is a mirror, reflecting every individual's deepest fears. AIDS is a magnet, indiscriminately attracting all manner of prejudices. AIDS is a juggernaut cutting a wide swath across the nation." AIDS has come to symbolize all manner of things, calling up prejudice in some individuals, accessing fears in others, and representing, at some level, our era's recognition that infectious diseases are not things of the past but the price we pay for living in a vital, constantly changing world.

The price is higher than many of us thought possible in an age of medical marvels, antibiotics, and vaccines (Morse, 1992). AIDS has struck hard at our people—and our illusions. Not long after experts concluded that the battle against infectious disease had been won and epidemics had ceased to be a significant factor in human life, AIDS struck, exacting a heavy toll from people and families, and decimating communities. Consider that:

• More than 30 million people worldwide are living with the human immunodeficiency virus (HIV) or with AIDS (Nathanson & Auerbach, 1999). AIDS is the deadliest sexually transmitted disease ever to confront humankind and ranks in severity with the Black Death that devastated Europe in the 14th century. In South Africa alone, AIDS is expected to kill six times as many people as were killed by atomic bombs in Hiroshima and Nagasaki. But, unlike a nuclear explosion, "there is no sound, no searing heat, no mushroom cloud, no buildings reduced to rubble. Just one mute death after another" (Sternberg, 1999a, p. 1D).

• Every day, 16,000 individuals, some of them young children, become infected with the virus. Sixteen million people are estimated to have died from AIDS, and the number is growing (Altman, 1999c; Bloom, 1998). Most of the infections occur in sub-Saharan Africa and Southeast Asia, as well as in impoverished communities in the United States and Europe. The long, uncompromising hands of Fate have left many of these people with a death sentence.

1

• In the United States, the epidemic has had devastating effects on gay and bisexual men, injecting drug users, and poor urban minorities. New infections of the virus that causes AIDS are "dangerously high" among minority gay men and African American and Latina heterosexual women (Steinhauer, 1999). More than 700,000 AIDS cases have been reported to the Centers for Disease Control (CDC) and Prevention. More than 420,000 people have died of AIDS, making it the fifth-leading cause of death in the United States among people ages 25 to 44 (CDC, 1999a).

• Young middle-class American high school and college students are sexually active, participating frequently in unprotected sex. In certain cases, the consequences are deadly. Several years ago a 20-year-old New York man with HIV infected at least 10 teenage girls with the AIDS virus (Barron, 1997). The man charmed the women or offered them drugs in exchange for sex, never telling them he was infected with HIV.

These examples and numerical estimates of AIDS deaths do not reveal the human side of the epidemic—sons and brothers who die young; wives and sisters who are plucked away before promising careers can begin; dads and moms who leave children to strangers; people with feelings, needs, and favorite hobbies like baseball, skydiving, or camping who pass away after years of struggle, leaving loved ones with memories and a life-long job of constructing explanations.

AIDS is the ultimate modern tragedy, a worldwide epidemic—pandemic— that has marched on, "exacting a deadly toll," leaving in its wake "decimated families, friendship networks, and entire communities" (Bailey, 1995, p. 210). Although new drugs have been developed that prolong the life of those infected with HIV, they do not work for everyone, are not accessible to all, and cannot prevent death once full-blown AIDS has been diagnosed. Even today, in an era of great medical discovery, the best hope for AIDS prevention lies in education, communication, and persuasion—in teaching people how HIV is transmitted, counseling them on steps they can take to protect themselves from contracting the virus, and convincing them that they must change their attitudes toward drugs and alluring, but dangerous, romantic liaisons.

Health policy expert Jaime Sepulveda expressed this simply: "AIDS is completely preventable with adequate information and the adoption of appropriate measures . . . [T]he often repeated dictum that education is the most effective weapon to prevent infection remains valid" (Sepulveda, Fineberg, & Mann, 1992, pp. 17,18). The key, in a word, is *persuasion.*

This book examines how we can apply persuasion theory and research to AIDS prevention. It focuses on ways to change attitudes and behaviors regarding HIV/AIDS, particularly unsafe sex. It explores how we can persuade people—people engaged in risky activities in American communities, those at risk in Third World countries, people different from you, or maybe you—to rethink attitudes toward sex and HIV. I call on theory and research in social psychology, communication, public health, and cultural anthropology to shed light on why people practice unsafe sex. I draw on theories to suggest the most effective ways to help people change HIV-related attitudes and behaviors, to discuss the impact of communication campaigns on safer sex practices, and to propose new methods to reduce stigmatized attitudes toward persons with AIDS.

This is fundamentally a book about AIDS prevention and persuasion. It is also a text that shows how practitioners can harness theories and research for the social good—particularly to alleviate daunting problems in health psychology and communication. This book is specifically designed to accomplish the following:

1. Show how theory can shed light on people's attitudes and interpersonal communication about an important health topic.
2. Help increase understanding of why people do not always take necessary precautions against HIV infection, and do not practice safer sex.
3. Suggest ways to use communication to change AIDS prevention behaviors.
4. Describe the many faces of HIV infection, the human side, cultural dimensions, and emotional hang-ups that act as barriers to safer sex.
5. Help you better understand your own attitudes toward AIDS prevention, perceptions of HIV infection, and feelings toward persons with AIDS.

AIDS AND HIV INFECTION

What is AIDS? What is HIV? Before discussing persuasion and HIV/AIDS prevention, it is important to understand these terms. People frequently confuse HIV and AIDS. HIV stands for the *human immunodeficiency virus,* an infinitesimally small infective agent tinier than a single cell. The HIV is especially troublesome because it infects white blood cells that are responsible for protecting the body against viral infections. The virus, James Slaff and John Brubaker (1985) note, "is a tiny killing machine of almost unbelievable durability and potency. . . . Once inside a body, it cannot be killed by any known medical means. It can launch a preemptive strike on the immune system, which is the body's way of defending itself from *all kinds* of germs" (p. 10).

AIDS, or *acquired immune deficiency syndrome,* is a larger medical condition, a series of illnesses that occur when the immune system has become disabled and unable to ward off infections (Kalichman, 1996). While some researchers argue that additional viruses are involved and that the epidemiology differs for different groups (Green, 1999; Root-Bernstein, 1993), the consensus is that HIV causes AIDS or is an important precursor. Thus, AIDS is typically the final stage of HIV infection. It occurs when the person's immune system has become disabled by HIV or other viruses, rendering it helpless against such life-threatening illnesses as skin cancer, parasitic infections, and infections of the nervous system.

An individual can be infected with HIV—or be HIV-positive—and not have AIDS. Magic Johnson is HIV-positive and does not have AIDS. Some people are infected with HIV but have not contracted AIDS because new drugs have prevented further damage to their immune systems. Although the drugs do not work for all individuals and can have serious side effects, they can postpone or perhaps prevent the onset of full-blown AIDS. Thus, an HIV infection does not lead immediately to AIDS. It typically takes between 2 to 15 years (usually about 10) for a person infected with HIV to contract AIDS (Rushing, 1995; see Fig. 1.1). The sooner HIV is caught, the sooner the person can be placed on drugs (protease inhibitors) to help forestall or prevent the onset of AIDS. That is why HIV testing is so important.

I say it "typically" takes between 2 and 15 years for an HIV-infected person to get AIDS because much depends on the nature of the individual's immune system and the HIV strain he or she has contracted. Some HIV-infected people (a small minority) never get AIDS; their immune systems are strong enough to fight it off. Because of these complications, experts frequently refer to the disease generically as HIV/AIDS.

HIV infection occurs when an infected individual's blood or other bodily fluid (e.g., semen) slips into another individual's bloodstream (Rushing, 1995). HIV is a blood-borne virus that cannot be contracted through casual contact with an infected person. It is not an ordinary infectious disease. As William Rushing notes:

> HIV is not transmitted through the air, like the microbes in tuberculosis and influenza. It cannot be transmitted through physical touch, like many fungal infec-

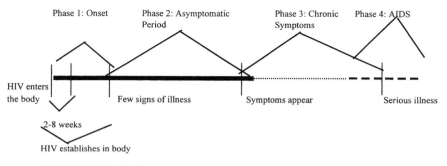

FIG. 1.1.   Early, middle, and late stages of HIV infection. From *Answering Your Questions About AIDS* (p. 31), by S. C. Kalichman, 1996, Washington, DC: APA.

tions are. It is not transmitted in contaminated water and food, like cholera, dysentery, and typhoid fever. . . . In sum, HIV cannot be transmitted through casual contact . . . and is not easy to "catch" or "pick up." It almost always requires the active participation of an individual in activity in which body fluid is exchanged with one or more persons. (p. 4)

HIV infection can occur in a number of ways, but the virus is most frequently transmitted through sex—heterosexual and homosexual (male to male) intercourse. It is also transmitted through sharing HIV-infected syringes (see Box 1.1).

Risk for HIV, Seth Kalichman (1996) reminds us, "is not as much a matter of who a person is as what a person does" (p. 105). In the United States, people are at high risk if they fall into the following categories:

- Men who have unprotected anal intercourse with other men.
- People who have shared needles, syringes, or other equipment to inject drugs.

BOX 1.1

A KNOWLEDGE TEST OF AIDS RISKS

Listed here are 10 questions to assess practical knowledge of AIDS transmission and prevention. Taking the test will enhance your knowledge of AIDS risks and help you understand how researchers tap this variable. (The questions are taken from Kelly, 1995, pp. 44–47.) Answers are given at the end.

1. You can get the virus that causes AIDS by:
   a. kissing an infected person
   b. having sexual intercourse with an infected person
   c. sharing the same water glass as an infected person
   d. being sneezed or coughed on
2. The AIDS virus is concentrated in:
   a. blood
   b. semen
   c. vaginal secretions
   d. all of the above
3. People who can transmit the AIDS virus to others:
   a. usually look sick
   b. will usually tell you they have the AIDS virus
   c. often look and feel completely healthy
   d. often don't know they even have it
   e. both c and d are correct

(Box Continues)

BOX 1.1 (Continued)

4. You can get AIDS from someone if:
   a. you have sex with them
   b. you share a drug-injecting needle with them
   c. you live in the same apartment building
   d. both a and b are correct

5. Which of the following steps reduces your risk for getting AIDS?:
   a. having sex only with a male (if you are a woman)
   b. having sex only with a female (if you are a man)
   c. using condoms during sex if you or your partner have had other sexual partners

6. What kind of condoms offers the best protection against AIDS?:
   a. natural skin condoms (made of animal skin)
   b. latex condoms

7. Men who have anal intercourse without a condom are:
   a. much more likely to contract the AIDS virus than men who don't have anal sex
   b. not very likely to contract the AIDS virus
   c. at little risk as long as they don't have anonymous partners
   d. at little risk as long as they don't have anal sex often

8. A person used to inject or "shoot" drugs but no longer does. Sex with this person would be:
   a. risky because many drug injectors have the AIDS virus.
   b. not very risky so long as the person doesn't use drugs now
   c. not very risky *unless* the person were also gay
   d. both b and c are correct

9. The best thing to use to clean needles (works) is:
   a. tap water
   b. Coca-Cola
   c. soapy water
   d. full-strength bleach
   e. all of the above are good to use

10. Someone who injects drugs:
    a. can potentially get the AIDS virus from partners who share needles
    b. can give the AIDS virus to his or her sexual partner
    c. can have (or father) a child born with the AIDS virus if infected with the AIDS virus
    d. should practice safer sex
    e. all of the above

Answers

1.) b; 2.) d; 3.) e; 4.) d; 5.) c; 6.) b; 7.) a; 8.) a; 9.) d; 10.) e

• Men or women who have had unprotected sexual intercourse with an injecting drug user.

People are at lower but considerable potential risk if they are

• heterosexually active, have sexually transmitted diseases (STDs), and have unprotected sex with many different people. Young people's risk level rises if they have sex with high-risk partners, such as homeless or runaway youths.

Risk groups for HIV differ, depending on the culture and the way the virus has spread. In the United States, the virus has been spread primarily through male-to-male sexual intercourse and injection drug use. In Africa, the virus is spread through heterosexual sex, and affluent heterosexual men and women are among its many victims. In Southeast Asia, the main mode of transmission is also heterosexual sex. Commercial sex workers are particularly apt to contract—and spread—the virus in Asian countries, notably Vietnam and Thailand.

BIOLOGY MEETS CULTURE

All this raises important questions: How did it happen? How could it occur? How could humanity, with all its sophistication and smarts, have fallen prey to a virus of such deadly proportions? How indeed, in our own era, characterized by medical marvels and technological mastery? The HIV virus that causes AIDS has existed since the early 1950s, perhaps for decades longer. Some researchers speculate that the virus spread from chimpanzees to humans living in Africa when people killed the animals for food.

The first report of AIDS-related symptoms in the United States came in February 1952 when a 28-year-old Tennessee man fell ill, caught pneumonia, and experienced all the debilitating infections now associated with AIDS, ultimately dying of them (Rotello, 1997). But his infection did not spread to others because the cultural mechanisms were not then in place. A rare virus, the HIV was of little interest because it was not capable of infecting an entire population.

For the virus to grow to epidemic proportions, a series of cultural changes had to occur, which would ensure that masses of people could be exposed. By an odd quirk of fate, this is precisely what occurred during the 1960s and 1970s. During this period of social upheaval, a number of events transpired that created just the kinds of nurturing environments in which the HIV could survive and prosper. During this two-decade period, writer Gabriel Rotello (1997) reminds us, society experienced "a revolution in the use of blood transfusions and blood products, an explosion in the use of injection drugs, a sexual revolution, (and) a gay revolution." These changes, Rotello notes, "brought about new global ecosystems in which the blood and sexual fluids of millions of people flowed into one another, and flowed the way HIV likes to travel: nonstop, straight to the vein" (pp. 20–21).

And so we return to the question: How did it happen? Who started the epidemiological fire? No one knows for sure. Rotello speculates that an adventure-seeking man from this or another country who carried the deadly microbe excitedly entered the exploding gay sex scene in San Francisco, shared heroin needles in New York, or otherwise mixed his infections "in a vast communal pool." Others argue that Haitians working in Africa got AIDS from Africans and infected Americans who were touring Haiti (Umeh, 1997). Whatever the mechanism, the handwriting was inscribed on the wall in June 1981. It was then that the CDC issued a strange report, noting that five young homosexual men had an unusual pneumonia that typically occurs only in individuals whose immune systems have been severely damaged. Over the next several months, the disease was found in other gay men, injecting drug users (IDUs), Haitians living in the United States, and recipients of blood transfusions. During this period, biology met culture and created an ecological change that has wreaked destruction ever since.

Several critical sociological factors made this possible. First, in the 1960s, the old blood transfusion method of transferring blood from one donor to one recipient was replaced by a more efficient method, whereby blood products were culled from multiple donors. With blood flowing into the United States from developing countries and international exchange of blood proliferating in the 1970s, it became possible for HIV-infected blood to get mixed into the mass blood pool. It turns out that this transmission route has not amplified the rate of HIV infection much, with one exception: hemophiliacs, who have become infected through transfusions. However, because there are only 15,000 hemophiliacs in the United States, blood transfusions account for only about 3% of all U.S. AIDS cases (Rotello, 1997).

A second factor is more important—changes in drug injection techniques. Although heroin and cocaine have been around for years, it has only been over the past 30 years that drug users began to inject drugs. They previously swallowed or sniffed their stuff (Rotello, 1997). Nowadays, drug users cluster together in *shooting galleries*—abandoned buildings or apartments—share needles, clean them in a common water cup, and draw blood from the needle while shooting up. Needle sharing is commonplace because it is convenient and strengthens emotional bonds among people frequently cut off from human affection. Unfortunately, this sharing provides just the type of access to the human body that facilitates the spread of the HIV. An HIV-infected person's blood can enter another drug user's bloodstream from the contaminated water or needle. And it frequently has.

The third factor precipitating change was sexual—liberalizing of sexual standards and dramatic increases in sexual intercourse among heterosexuals across the globe. Approximately 50% of American teenagers have had sexual intercourse before the age of 18, with Blacks reporting more sexual experience than Whites (CDC, 2000; Jemmott & Jones, 1993). Many heterosexual young people are at risk for sexually transmitted diseases, which cause venereal sores that give the HIV access to the bloodstream. It is expected that there will be more cases of HIV among heterosexual American adolescents, although the dangers of hetero-sexual AIDS are actually greater in some African and Asian countries, where men regard it as their prerogative to have concubines, prostitution runs rampant, and venereal disease frequently goes untreated.

Unquestionably, the group most affected by expanding sexuality in the United States has been gay men. During the late 1960s and early 1970s, gay culture came out of the closet. And when it came out, it exploded with a bang. Or a series of big sexual bangs. Anal intercourse became particularly common-place, and this type of intercourse creates high risk because HIV-infected semen can easily penetrate the thin walls of the anus and rectum. To make matters worse, gay sex frequently occurred among closely knit core groups, such as those that hung out at city bathhouses. Men from these core groups then inter-mingled sexually with others in the gay population. As a result, STDs rapidly increased in these core groups, and diseases—notably HIV—spread like wild-fire through the gay population. "AIDS," Robert Root-Bernstein (1993) notes, "became a problem for homosexual men only when rampant promiscuity, fre-quent anal forms of intercourse, new and sometimes physically traumatic forms of sex, and the frequent concomitants of drug use and multiple concurrent in-fections paved the way" (pp. 291–292).

Society had somehow managed to create just the sort of conditions that fa-cilitated the epidemic spread of the HIV. As Root-Bernstein notes, "social revo-lutions always have medical consequences." Pooling of blood products, sharing of dirty needles, and most importantly, incredible increases in sex among strangers provided just the sorts of entries the HIV needed to the vast human ecological pool. A virus that required primarily sexual contact for transmission was in the right place at the right time—and, for the human race, the conse-quences were nothing short of tragic.

SAFER SEX, AIDS, AND PERSUASION

HIV is spread by sexual intercourse or by sharing infected needles to inject drugs. Sex is the most common transmission mode. But not all sex puts people at risk. People cannot contract the virus through sexual contact if semen, vaginal fluid, or blood are not exchanged. Thus, kissing, hugging, petting, and mutual masturbation are completely safe from HIV infection. They fall under the cate-gory of **safe sex**.

It is commonly believed that sex with condoms constitutes safe sex. How-ever, although such sex is relatively risk-free, it is not 100% without risk because condoms can occasionally break, or may be used incorrectly. **Safer sex** refers to sexual activities that greatly reduce the risk of HIV infection—primarily anal or vaginal sex performed with latex condoms.

As Kalichman (1996) notes, "condoms significantly reduce the risk for HIV infection during sexual intercourse. Research has shown that condoms made of latex do not allow HIV to pass through" (p. 206). For purposes of this book, **safer sex refers to anal or vaginal sexual intercourse performed with a latex condom.**

Obviously, the safest sexual practice is *all but intercourse,* or sex that stops short of intercourse. Given the upsurge in teenage sex since the 1960s, the large numbers of adolescents who have had sexual intercourse, and the problems that teenage sex presents for adolescents who are still maturing emotionally and mentally, there is little doubt that society would be better off if numerous high school students had less sex and postponed sexual intercourse until they were older and more mature. However admirable the goal, it is difficult to achieve in the United States and much of the world. In the United States, the media show sexual images repeatedly on prime time and in the afternoon (Greenberg & Busselle, 1996), a recent president of the United States admitted to having "sexual relations"—his words—with a woman young enough to be his daughter, and adolescence is frequently celebrated as an era in which young people use sex to establish autonomy from their elders. And this is just in the United States; many Third World countries are more sex-positive than the United States. In some African countries, polygamy is common. Thus, it is not easy to dissuade young adults from engaging in sex.

In this book, I take the position that safer sex constitutes a practical, highly effective method of HIV prevention. Some people will disagree with this position, claiming that condoms are immoral or encourage promiscuity. To those who say this, I reply: I understand your feelings and agree there are too many people having sex at too young an age. However, it is difficult to persuade people to "just say no" to sex when sex satisfies so many emotional needs. A more realistic goal—settling for half a loaf instead of a whole—is to persuade young people to engage in safer sex, that is, sexual activity that will at least protect them from HIV infection. Contrary to what some well-meaning conservatives believe, there is evidence that condom promotion campaigns do not increase sexual activity among adolescents (Sellers, McGraw, & McKinlay, 1994).

Others oppose safer sex education for a different reason: They believe that society has no business telling young people what to do with their bodies. Some gay activists make this point, arguing that the proscription that a gay man should use a condom every time he engages in any sexual activity "demands an unattainable standard of behavior" (Odets, 1995, p. 14). I respect this libertarian position. I agree that a society that coerces its members not to engage in sexual activities they find satisfying is a society that violates basic human liberties. However, things get complicated when an individual's desire to exercise his or her sexual liberties can lead to another person getting infected with HIV. Society has an interest in protecting public health, and this means we need to balance civil liberties with larger questions of the public good (Bayer, 1994; Etzioni, 1998). Recommending that people engage in safer sex, reinforcing them for doing so, and developing institutional safeguards to help people protect themselves and others strikes me as a reasonable way to balance individual rights and the social good.

The focus of this book is on persuading individuals to practice safer sex. Changing sexual behaviors is not the only way to use education to prevent the spread of AIDS. It is also important to persuade at-risk individuals to get tested for HIV or, in the case of injecting drug users, to use bleach to disinfect dirty needles. (Bleach kills the HIV.) As new anti-AIDS drugs become more effective and an HIV vaccine is someday developed that prevents infection, persuasion efforts will revolve around convincing individuals to regularly take medications and to get their HIV shot. As of now, these events are not on the horizon. Thus, the focus of the book is on the age-old problem of convincing people to temper their impulses, reign in their desires, develop the self-control needed to say no to risky sex, and to acquire the ability to effectively practice safer sex. It is also about the larger issue of persuading individuals to view with more empathy and compassion those who have contracted AIDS.

Persuasion Terminology

This is a book about persuasion and AIDS prevention. I've introduced the latter, but not the former. Contrary to popular opinion, persuasion does not mean influence by force. That is more akin to coercion, which occurs when, for example, a prisoner of war condemns the United States in public because his captors are holding a gun to his head. Coercion also occurs when an influence agent has undermined a person's freedom or destroyed his or her autonomy, as has occurred in religious cults (Perloff, 1993). This is not the same as persuasion.

Persuasion requires that individuals the persuader is trying to influence have free choice or perceive that they have free choice. What's more, persuasion never involves a communicator forcing a view on someone else or injecting the other person with a message like a doctor injects a vaccine through a needle. Instead, persuasion always involves the persuader convincing message recipients to change their own mind about the topic. Persuasion is self-persuasion. Persuaders persuade us to change our minds, feelings, or behaviors. They provide the arguments. They set up the bait. We make the change—so we are responsible for what we do or don't do. This is especially true in the case of AIDS preventive communications, which call to mind strong feelings about sex, are strongly connected with our relationships—with wives, husbands, and lovers— and conjure up myths, hang-ups and prejudice. It is not easy to persuade people about AIDS. People do not start out with a blank slate. That is why so many studies have been conducted, theories are invoked, and I devote an entire book to understanding why people resist safer sex persuasion and how we can use research to help surmount the barriers.

Research Shortcomings and Strengths

The chapters in this book call on research, particularly on sex. Research plays a critical role in helping to explain why people practice unsafe sex and in suggesting preventive strategies. But research is not infallible. Studies of sexual behavior rely on self-reports of risky sex. People don't always tell the truth when it comes to sex. They brag about how often they have unsafe sex or underestimate how many times they use a condom. Or they may not accurately recall what they did and when they did it (Catania et al., 1990). Telephone surveys may misrepresent people's sexual practices by using words like "vaginal intercourse," "anal intercourse," or other terms that respondents find difficult to understand (Binson & Catania, 1998). Some respondents may be offended by this language and hang up on interviewers.

The upshot is that we should view research with a healthy skepticism, remembering that we are using imperfect methods to extract highly sensitive information from people. Our results are not the gospel truth, and they will change over time and as new procedures for probing sexual behavior are developed. However, systematic, theory-oriented research provides new facts, ideas, and insights about why people do or don't engage in HIV-prevention behaviors. Research also provides important clues about how to use persuasive communication to promote healthier HIV-prevention attitudes and actions.

WHAT COMES NEXT

In the chapters that follow, I discuss AIDS, safer sex, and persuasion. I present research and theory, hopefully in a way that will turn students on to social science and help them appreciate its practical benefits. Given the sheer number of articles on AIDS that are published each year, I have opted to limit my scope, focusing attention on AIDS prevention in the United States.

The next chapter introduces the ways in which cognitive theories have been applied to HIV prevention. Chapter 3 continues this discussion, focusing on other social psychological theories of attitudes, and interpersonal communication. Interpersonal communication about sex is pivotal because talking can do so much to overcome people's resistance to safer sex practices. Both of these chapters feature safer sex snapshots—interviews in which young people talk honestly about sex and safer sex. The first snapshot appears in Box 1.2.

Chapter 4 looks at culture and AIDS prevention. I examine why ethnic minorities, low-income women, and so many people from the African continent

BOX 1.2

SAFER SEX SNAPSHOT

What do young people really think about safer sex? What's their view of condoms and sex in the age of AIDS? Mark Fritz, a skilled interviewer with a background in the health sciences, set out to answer these questions by talking with heterosexual and gay young adults. Fritz's interviews appear in a series of boxed sections in this chapter and the ones that follow. In the interview, *I* refers to interviewer and *R* to respondent. This interview is with a 24-year-old White female undergraduate at an Ohio university.

I: Are you sexually active?

R: I think that you would have to define what sexually active means. I mean, Bill Clinton [had] a tough time defining it and he [was] President!

I: Let's define sexual activity as any intimate interaction between people where the exchange of bodily fluids took place.

R: Well, that certainly limits the things I would have considered. However, under your definition, I will say yes.

I: Have you demanded the use of condoms with your sexual partner?

R: I try not to be that demanding about my partner using any kind of protection. I am on the pill so I feel that there is no need to break the magic of the moment by injecting some secondary demand that probably will be ignored anyway.

I: When was the last time you had sexual relations?

R: He took me to the (Cleveland) Indians game Saturday and then we went to dinner. After we got back to his place, we made love. It was nice.

I: How do you feel about condom use in general?

R: Whatever floats your boat.

I: How do you think your partner feels about condom use?

R: He hates them and frankly, I can't blame him. For me it certainly puts a crimp on what I would like to do to satisfy him.

I: Why do you use condoms?

R: I don't really ask my partners to use a rubber and except for one guy I dated a while ago, have never had sex while using one. However, the one guy I did date used them because he was scared of contracting AIDS. His paranoia had an impact on our relationship too. I broke up with him because he couldn't seem to get it out of his head that I didn't sleep around and, therefore, didn't carry a risk for him of getting AIDS. A real weirdo!

I: Do you carry condoms with you when you go out?

R: That is a very good question because, actually, I have one here in my purse. I have carried it for a long time and don't know if it would actually work or

(Box continues)

BOX 1.2 (*Continued*)

not now. In fact, it has been banged around so much it probably has some kind of expiration date on the package that would tell me to throw it out. With all the shit I carry in my purse, it probably has holes in it.

COMMENT: This woman is honest and open about her sexual feelings, which is great. However, she is extremely reluctant to propose condom use. Like many young women, she is afraid of alienating her male lover, places satisfying him ahead of her own health, and seems to lack confidence in her ability to discuss condoms. She might benefit from some of the safer sex communication strategies discussed in chapter 5.

---

engage in risky activities. Rather than criticizing folks, I try to look at things from their perspective, attempting to understand the psychology behind their decisions to practice unsafe sex and the reasons their sexual communication is not as effective as it might be.

The first four chapters help lay the foundation for understanding why people do not always harbor positive attitudes toward safer sex and AIDS prevention, and why they fail to take needed precautions.

Building on these foundations, the next two chapters outline theory-based strategies for persuading people to take sexual precautions. Chapter 5 examines major social psychological theories of persuasion, looking at ways to use the communicator and message to convince people to protect themselves against HIV. Chapter 6 adopts a more macro approach, examining diffusion and social marketing theories and reviewing different campaigns directed at risk groups. I end the book by examining why people stigmatize persons with AIDS and how to use persuasion to reduce AIDS stigma.

This is a book that applies theory and research to a vexing social issue and the most basic of human desires. I hope it increases your insights into AIDS prevention and gives you more understanding of your own attitudes toward HIV and persons with AIDS.

CHAPTER TWO

Cognitive Foundations of AIDS Prevention Behavior

This chapter and the one that follows introduce theories of AIDS preventive behavior. The emphasis on the word "theory" may throw students for a loop. Theories call up negative images in many people's minds. What do you think when you see the word *theory?* Do you think of scientific formulas, jargon-filled books, and boring discussions? I did when I first encountered the term in graduate courses. "Why are these books so unpleasant to read?" I thought. "Why do they use all these strange-sounding words that have little to do with real life?"

I changed my mind the more I read. As I pored over book chapters and journal articles, I found my mind buzzing, stimulated by how theory could shed light on everyday situations at home and work. I slowly realized that scholars were using words differently than I had as an undergraduate, yet were unpeeling provocative layers of life. Theory, I learned, isn't an enemy but a friend, a way to help you understand and cope better with life.

Theory plays a critical role in social science because it generates ideas. These ideas can then be tested empirically—by scientific rules of inquiry—to see if they are right or wrong. The facts—or findings as we call them—that emerge from empirical research yield insights, help people solve personal problems, and even point toward new pathways to rectify social wrongs. The best theories are those that accurately predict human behavior and suggest how to create more humane ways for people to live their lives.

At some level, everyone has theories or higher order beliefs about the world that guide their everyday decisions. You may have a theory about what causes relationships to sour, or how to harness skills and ambitions to achieve career success, or how to lose weight. "Everyone forms theories (mental models) to explain what they have observed," notes psychologist Donald Norman (1988). He cautions that "mental models are often constructed from fragmentary evidence, with but a poor understanding of what is happening, and with a kind of naive psychology that postulates causes, mechanisms, and relationships even when there are none" (pp. 38–39). So it is with AIDS.

Many intuitive theories of AIDS prevention are constructed from inaccurate notions of the risk of HIV infection. For example, college students frequently use simple rules—or primitive theories—to judge the riskiness of sex partners. According to Sunyna Williams and her colleagues (1992), students "tend to assume that risky people are those who dress provocatively, whom one met in bars, who were older than most college students, who are from large cities, or are overly anxious for sex" (p. 926). The problem with this "theory" is that it's based on stereotypes and gross generalizations. "Because the only way to accurately determine someone's AIDS risk is through knowledge of that person's HIV status," Williams and her associates note, "the use of any other cues to assess risk will often provide a dangerous, false sense of security" (p. 927). An elaborate scientific theory of AIDS risk offers a broader, more comprehensive view. It would tell who is at risk and why. A psychological theory of people's judgments might tell why people tend to use stereotypes in judging sexual riskiness rather than factual information. As researcher Laura Leviton (1989) notes, "formal scientific theories may help to counteract mistaken beliefs about AIDS prevention" (p. 43).

Theories can also help practitioners develop more effective campaigns to prevent the spread of AIDS. Not realizing theories are available to guide them, campaigners often rely on trendy ideas or gut instincts. Typically fuzzy entities, gut instincts usually aren't written down. They lack clarity and explanatory power. Gut instincts are rarely tested empirically, so one doesn't know if they work or are just a lucky rabbit's foot to be massaged before a decision. By contrast, formal scientific theories afford a more elaborate way to design a campaign. They aren't based solely on intuitive judgments. They define terms, contain concepts, propose linkages between variables, and make predictions (Hage, 1972). Predictions can be stated formally and tested to see if they accurately forecast reality. Moreover, because they are formally articulated and published in scientific journals, theories and the research they generate can be reviewed by colleagues and revised by dissenting scholars. The revision process can generate new theories and research, which may suggest better ways of helping people cope with life's dilemmas.

Now that the "T" word is out on the table, let's explore different theories of AIDS prevention behavior. This chapter, focusing on psychological foundations, examines cognitive decision theories. Chapter 3 then takes a broader look at the underpinnings of AIDS attitudes and behaviors, examining other social psychological approaches, as well as communication perspectives.

OVERVIEW OF COGNITIVE DECISION THEORIES

Cognitive decision theories assume that people are rational creatures who consider the costs and benefits of alternatives and make careful use of information available to them. Theorists assume that people weigh expected costs against expected benefits and make decisions based on what they think will best serve their self-interest and personal well-being (Leviton, 1989). When it comes to safer sex, cognitive decision scholars argue that people size up the risks of getting involved with someone sexually, render a judgment about the effectiveness of protective actions, and make a decision on what they'll do in a given situation. Individuals may also consider the views of significant others, like friends and family. Since people make decisions based on the probabilities of X causing Y, theorists argue that it should be possible to model their behavior with scientific formulas. Although the theories differ in factors they emphasize (Weinstein, 1993), they share these similarities:

1. They are cognitive and place emphasis on people's **beliefs** about the consequences of performing a particular precautionary behavior.

2. They fall under the heading of **expectancy-value approaches** since they assume that behavior primarily depends on the person's beliefs (or expectations) that a particular action will produce a particular outcome, and the value the person places on the outcome.

3. They focus on mental processes that underlie people's decisions to perform one or another social behavior.

4. They place a premium on self-interest. The theories assume, in varying degrees, that you can motivate people to take action if you convince them that they will gain something by complying and lose by not complying. There is little emphasis on appealing to people's morals or obligations to their fellow human beings.

Two major cognitive decision theories are the theory of reasoned action (TRA; Azjen & Fishbein, 1980; Fishbein & Ajzen, 1975) and the health belief model (Becker, 1974; Becker & Rosenstock, 1987).

THEORY OF REASONED ACTION

What, you may ask, could a theory of reasoned action tell us about sex, which is not always reasoned but inevitably involves action?

It's a fair question. In fact, the TRA has many interesting implications for safer sex and AIDS prevention. Martin Fishbein and Icek Ajzen, who developed the approach, use the term *reasoned action* to describe the theory because they believe that most behavior is contemplated, or reasoned through, and under people's control.

The theory maintains that three factors govern performance of behavior: **intention, attitude toward the behavior, and subjective norm.** Intentions play a pivotal role. Intentions, Ajzen (1991) notes, "are assumed to capture the motivational factors that influence a behavior; they are indications of how hard people are willing to try, of how much of an effort they are planning to exert, in order to perform the behavior" (p. 181). Research shows that people usually— but not always—do what they intend to do.

Your attitude toward a behavior is your "judgment that performing the behavior is good or bad" (Ajzen & Fishbein, 1980, p. 6). Attitudes toward behavior consist of two elements: your *beliefs* about the consequences of putting the behavior into action, and *evaluations,* your feelings about these consequences. Beliefs are cognitive, evaluations affective.

Different beliefs are likely to be *salient* or personally significant. The salient beliefs—those that come immediately to people's minds when they think of the attitude—are the ones that figure most importantly in a person's attitude.

Subjective norm is a person's inclination to go along with the views of people he or she respects. It has two components: *normative beliefs,* or beliefs that people you respect recommend that you perform the behavior, and *motivation to comply,* your desire to go along with what these folks say.

The theory of reasoned action (TRA) is a linear model. Behavior is best predicted by intentions. Intentions are predicted by attitude and subjective norm. In certain situations, attitude will forecast intentions better; in other cases, pressure to go along with significant others will predict intentions more accurately (see Fig. 2.1). External factors, like a person's health history or cultural context, influence intentions by affecting attitudes and subjective norms.

The theory can help explain and predict AIDS preventive behavior. How do we test the theory's hypotheses about unsafe sex? We can't observe people in their bedrooms. Therefore, we must devise questionnaires that probe thoughts, feelings, and intentions. Let's say we want to predict whether a group of at-risk youngsters engage in unsafe sex. Just ask them, the practical side of us shouts. Not so fast, Martin Fishbein and Susan Middlestadt (1989) say; not so fast:

> There are many different behaviors that can be classified as "safe" or "unsafe" sex. It is thus possible for two people to define "unsafe" sex in very different ways. This being the case, asking a person whether he or she practices "safe" or "unsafe" sex is not very meaningful. For example, one person might assume that engaging in any type of intercourse without a condom is unsafe, while another may believe that this is true only with respect to anal intercourse. A third person may believe that condoms are necessary only when one doesn't know one's partner; and a fourth might believe that "unsafe" sex is defined as having sex with a gay male or a drug user. From the perspective of the medical community, all of these people may be engaging in high-risk sexual behaviors, yet all might report that they are practicing "safe" sex. (p. 97)

Maybe it seems strange to subject sex to such cognitive scrutiny, but people are complex mental and emotional creatures, as well as critters endowed with sex drives. Situations and people differ, and interpretations of safer sex differ dramatically. Fishbein argues that if you want to accurately forecast a particular behavior in a situation, you have to get down and be specific. Instead of asking

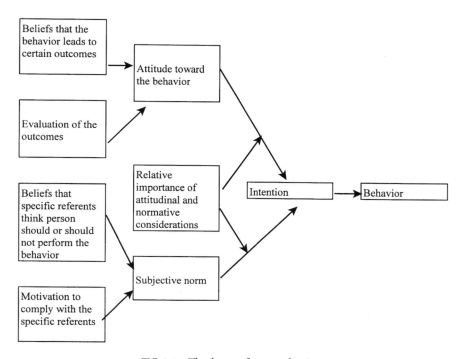

FIG. 2.1.   The theory of reasoned action.

"Do people practice safer sex?" he urged researchers to be more precise and consider four factors. The factors to consider when measuring safer sex are:

1. action (e.g., are you interested in knowing whether at-risk heterosexual men use a condom during anal sex, or vaginal sex, or alternatively if they purchase condoms at the drug store?).

2. target (are you interested in respondents' use of a latex or nonlatex condom?).

3. context (are you concerned with use of a condom with a long-term partner or a casual acquaintance?).

4. time (do you want to know whether an injecting drug user performs safer sex in the short term—a few days after a counseling session—or over the long haul, say, a 6-month period?).

Heterosexual Sex

Let's see how we might apply these principles to an actual situation. Suppose you want to explore one particular AIDS preventive activity: whether women

intend to tell their partners to always use a condom. This is an important behavior. Women can protect themselves against AIDS by insisting that partners
use a condom, but many may be afraid to ask their lovers. You decide you want
to learn why.

This is exactly what consumed Darius Chan and Martin Fishbein, who explored this issue some years ago. More than 300 college-age women filled out a
questionnaire that measured safer sex intentions, attitudes, norms, and beliefs.
The researchers used similar words for all questions to encourage respondents
to think of the same situation when answering the questions. Here are the ways
the researchers measured key variables in their study:

Intention:
   I will tell my partner to use a condom every time I have sexual intercourse.
$$7 \quad 6 \quad 5 \quad 4 \quad 3 \quad 2 \quad 1$$
                Likely   Unlikely

Attitude:
   My telling my partner to use a condom every time I have sexual intercourse is:
$$7 \quad 6 \quad 5 \quad 4 \quad 3 \quad 2 \quad 1$$
                Good   Bad

Subjective Norm:
   Most people who are important to me think I _____ tell my partner to use a condom every time I have sexual intercourse:
$$7 \quad 6 \quad 5 \quad 4 \quad 3 \quad 2 \quad 1$$
                Should   Should not

To explore foundations of attitude and subjective norm, Chan and Fishbein
asked participants other questions. For instance, they measured beliefs by asking respondents to judge how likely it was that certain outcomes would occur if
they told their partner to use a condom every time they had sexual intercourse.
As an example, respondents indicated whether telling a partner to use a condom would make their lover feel angry or make sex less intimate. Evaluations
were assessed by asking respondents how they felt about these outcomes. For
example, did they feel that their lover's anger about condom use was good
or bad?

Although the questions were personal, respondents filled out the surveys.
Chan and Fishbein (1993) discovered that attitude and subjective norm predicted women's intentions to tell their partners to use condoms every time they
had sexual intercourse. Women who had more favorable attitudes toward this
behavior and felt motivated to go along with significant others' recommendations intended to tell partners to use condoms. More interesting, those who did
not intend to tell a partner to use condoms harbored different beliefs than those

who intended to tell a partner to practice safer sex. Nonintenders were more apt to believe that telling a partner to use a condom would:

- "Cause conflict between me and my partner"
- "Make my partner angry"
- "Lead to loss of trust between me and my partner"
- "Make sex less intimate"
- "Decrease my partner's sexual pleasure"

This helps us understand why some women do not want to tell a partner to use a condom. They are fearful that conflict will erupt and sex will become less pleasurable.

Gay Sex

"Despite the fact that by now virtually everyone knows how AIDS is spread and how to avoid it," Gabriel Rotello (1997) observes, "it is continuing to saturate the gay male population at the same levels it always has" (p. 3). Concerned about the devastating effects AIDS has had on gay communities, researchers seized the opportunity to apply the TRA to gay men's sexual behaviors.

Fishbein and his colleagues (1992) studied gay men from different cities, including Albany and Seattle. Respondents answered a series of personal questions about their sexual attitudes and safer-sex intentions. They indicated their intentions to engage in insertive anal intercourse without exchanging semen, to allow their partners to come inside them during receptive anal intercourse, and to engage in receptive anal intercourse with their partners without a condom if the partners promised not to come inside them. These are risky behaviors, so it was important to pinpoint factors that influenced men's intentions to perform these actions.

Men who harbored positive attitudes toward these behaviors and believed that significant others felt they should perform them were likely to say they intended to engage in unsafe sex. Respondents' attitudes were important: Those men who felt that risky sex practices were good, safe, pleasant, and wise indicated they would be willing to take a chance. Why would men feel that sexual behaviors that could put them and their partners at risk are safe or wise? Why does the sheer pleasantness of the act outweigh more rational considerations? The theory doesn't answer these questions. But we get some guidance from the functional approach to attitudes (see chapter 3).

One other important finding emerged from Fishbein's study. The power of subjective norms depended on the city. Norms exerted the strongest impact on men's safer sex intentions in Seattle and had the smallest influence in Albany. Why might this be? Fishbein and his colleagues explained:

Seattle, the city for which normative influences were greatest, has a large and visible gay population. Gay organizations have long existed there and have been instrumental in securing strong antidiscrimination protection for the city's gay population. . . . Albany, on the other hand, has had no locally generated media campaigns to combat AIDS. The gay community in Albany is small, largely invisible, and blends into the general population. . . . It seems reasonable to conclude that the better organized the gay community, the more normative pressure influences the formation of intentions to engage (or to not engage) in risky sexual behaviors. A better organized community is more likely to develop prevention services and to provide a relatively well-linked interpersonal network which enhances interpersonal interactions. This may then lead to more interpersonal or social influence. (p. 1009)

Armed with this information, campaign specialists may opt to use different strategies to change safer sex behaviors in Albany than in Seattle. One strategy will not fit all. This point, which is taken up in chapter 6, came from theory, specifically the theory of reasoned action.

HEALTH BELIEF MODEL

Like other cognitive decision theories, the Health Belief Model (HBM) assumes that people are motivated to protect their health and they make rational calculations of costs and benefits before adopting precautionary behavior (Carmel, 1991). As the name implies, the HBM assigns a central role to beliefs—specifically, beliefs about the threat of a particular disease and ways of coping with the illness. In the classic formulation of the model, theorists identified four types of health beliefs:

1. Perceived susceptibility, the person's perception of the chances of contracting the disease.
2. Perceived severity, assessments of consequences of the health threat.
3. Perceived benefits, beliefs about the effectiveness of various coping actions.
4. Perceived barriers, perceptions of the negative consequences of coping actions.

The first two beliefs—perceived susceptibility and perceived severity—focus on the threat posed by disease. The second two center on coping responses. The model assumes that social and demographic factors influence health beliefs, beliefs trigger a motivation for health-protective action, and cues in the social environment lead to action (see Fig. 2.2).

Health beliefs about AIDS preventive behavior have been usefully measured by Matthew Zagumny and D. Brian Brady (1998). The following are sample items from their AIDS health belief scale.

Perceived susceptibility:

I am afraid that I might contract AIDS.

            1   2   3   4   5   6
        Strongly disagree   Strongly agree

Perceived severity:

I would rather have any other terminal illness than AIDS.

            1   2   3   4   5   6
        Strongly disagree   Strongly agree

Perceived benefits:

If a condom is not available, it would be worth the effort to discontinue sexual activity to obtain a condom.

            1   2   3   4   5   6
        Strongly disagree   Strongly agree

Perceived barriers:

Using a condom seems like an insult to my partner.

            1   2   3   4   5   6
        Strongly disagree   Strongly agree

Research indicates that AIDS health beliefs are important factors in safer-sex decision making (Aspinwall et al., 1991; Bryan et al., 1997; Hingson et al., 1990;

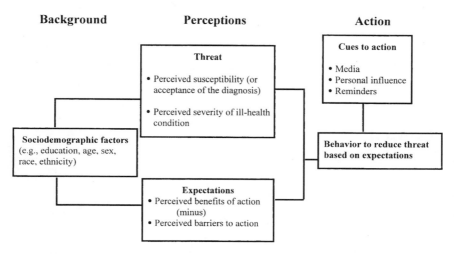

FIG. 2.2. The Health Belief Model. Adapted from "The health belief model and HIV risk behavior change" (p. 11), by I. M. Rosenstock, V. J. Strecher, and M. H. Becker. In R. J. DiClemente and J. L. Peterson (Eds.), *Preventing AIDS: Theories and Methods of Behavioral Interventions,* 1994, New York: Plenum.

Mattson, 1999; Wulfert & Wan, 1995). Perceived barriers or drawbacks of condom use can be particularly significant predictors of HIV risk reduction behavior (Gillespie, 1997). Several perceived drawbacks have emerged from research, including (a) identity stigma ("Men who suggest using a condom are really boring"), (b) embarrassment about negotiation and use ("I never know what to say when my partner and I need to talk about condoms or other protection"), and (c) embarrassment about purchase ("It would be embarrassing to be seen buying condoms in a store") (Helweg-Larsen & Collins, 1994, p. 228). If people are more persuaded by disadvantages like these than by advantages of using condoms, chances are they won't perform safer sex that often.

The HBM assists in understanding why many young people frequently engage in unsafe sex (Kalichman, 1998). The perceived drawbacks of condom use —embarrassment and lack of pleasure—are salient and come quickly to mind. The perceived benefits are harder to visualize. As Everett Rogers (1995) notes, the unwanted event that has been avoided "is difficult to perceive because it is a non-event, the absence of something that otherwise might have happened. For example, an individual's not contracting HIV/AIDS is invisible, unobservable, and hence difficult or impossible to comprehend" (p. 217).

The HBM has advanced knowledge about AIDS preventive behaviors; yet, like all theories it has limits. The model doesn't make precise predictions about the impact of health beliefs on behavior. Instead, as Weinstein (1993) observes, it "is more accurately described as a short list of variables than as a theoretical model" (p. 327). In addition, one of the key components of the model—perceived susceptibility—has proved more elusive and complex than researchers assumed. The model assumes that people recognize when they are susceptible to a health threat and take steps to protect themselves from danger. The problem is that we don't always do this, particularly with regard to AIDS. In the next section, I discuss how people frequently deny their vulnerability to AIDS threats. I focus on beliefs of college students, adopting a folksier approach to help readers grapple with these issues.

The Illusion of Invulnerability

"I never thought I needed to worry about AIDS," confessed Jana Brent. "I thought it only happened to big-city people, not people like me who are tucked away in the Midwest. But 18 months ago, I was diagnosed with the virus that causes AIDS. Now I live in fear of this deadly illness every single day of my life," Jana told a writer from *Cosmopolitan* (Ziv, 1998).

Born in Great Bend, Kansas, Jana had an unhappy childhood: broken home, deadbeat dad, life in foster homes. After moving to Kansas City and completing vocational training, Jana met Sean, a good-looking 22-year-old, who flattered her with compliments, told her he loved her, and seemed like the answer to her prayers. They soon became sexually intimate. "We had sex, on average, four times a week," Jana recalls. "We didn't talk about using condoms or getting tested, and I wasn't worried about using protection. We used condoms only when we had any lying around." Fearing Jana might get pregnant, Sean coaxed her into having anal sex, which they performed 10 times, never with a condom.

One day in July, Jana decided to get an AIDS test. The test confirmed her worst fears: She was HIV-positive and had been infected by Sean. He had tested positive years earlier, but never bothered to tell Jana. Although she knew the dangers of unprotected sex, Jana felt invulnerable. "I was one of those girls who thought, *AIDS won't happen to me,*" she said (p. 241).

What crosses your mind when you read this story? That it's sad and tragic? That Jana took risks, ones your friends or you wouldn't take? That she's not like you, with her checkered past and desperate need for companionship?

Perhaps you didn't have such thoughts at all—but if you did, if you tried to psychologically distance yourself from Jana or told yourself her situation is *much* different from yours or silently whispered "this couldn't happen to me because . . . ," you've revealed something important. You've shown yourself a mite susceptible to what psychologists call **the illusion of invulnerability.**

What is the illusion of invulnerability? It is people's belief—or need to believe—that bad things won't happen to them. "People tend to think they are invulnerable," Neil Weinstein (1980) notes. "They expect others to be victims of misfortune, not themselves. Such ideas imply not merely a hopeful outlook on life, but an error of judgment that can be labeled *unrealistic optimism*" (p. 806). People assume they are less likely than others to fall prey to diseases, such as lung cancer and heart disease, and believe they are less apt to experience an array of negative outcomes, including divorce, drinking problems, and getting fired from a job (e.g., Weinstein, 1980).

We—all of us—cling to such illusions for many reasons. We are defensive. We need to protect ourselves from knowledge that could threaten our ability to function in everyday life and might undermine our self-confidence. So we erect psychological shields around ourselves—denial, defensiveness, distortion. We tell ourselves that we're invulnerable to negative outcomes—we're stronger, healthier, and more resilient than the average Joe or Jane.

We have also learned to be unrealistically optimistic. We're in touch with our own psyches and are cognizant of our physical and mental abilities. Lacking knowledge of other people, we assume they're weaker or more vulnerable. The mass media also feed our biases. Because the media love sensational stories about people who fall off cliffs or die of cancer at a young age or get divorced within days of their marriage, we conclude that many other people are "like that," weak or prone to misfortune. We rely on *the representativeness heuristic,* or psychological rule of thumb that says you assign a person to a particular category based on whether the individual's characteristics resemble the typical member of the category.

The representativeness heuristic helps people maintain their illusions of invulnerability. "If they do not see themselves as fitting the stereotype," Weinstein (1980) notes, "the representativeness heuristic suggests that people will conclude that the event will not happen to them, overlooking the possibility that few of the people who experience the event may actually fit the stereotype" (p. 808).

How forcefully the illusion of invulnerability operates in the arena of HIV/AIDS! The rate of HIV infection has risen sharply among young people (DiClemente, 1992a). Sexually transmitted diseases are common among adolescents (about one in every seven reports an STD), and the presence of STDs increases susceptibility to HIV. Yet college students perceive they are less susceptible to HIV infection than other persons; they underestimate their own susceptibility to HIV, while overestimating other students' risk (Mickler, 1993; Seal & Agostinelli, 1996). Although teenagers and college students are knowledgeable about AIDS and AIDS prevention strategies, the majority do not see themselves at risk for HIV, and few report an intention of getting tested for the virus (Brenders & Garrett, 1993; Fisher & Fisher, 1996; Freimuth, Edgar, & Hammond, 1987). (See Safer Sex Snapshot, Box 2.1.)

One factor that feeds perceptions of invulnerability is the representative heuristic. Barbara Kaplan and Vivian Shayne (1993) perceptively note:

> With the emphasis on injecting drug abusers and homosexual men as high-risk groups, many heterosexuals and homosexuals with a limited number of partners are likely to decide that they are at negligible risk, that is, that they themselves do not "match" the high-risk population. News stories of prominent and not-so-prominent people with AIDS have often focused on members of high-risk groups, so that in considering the probability statistics for AIDS (e.g., that it is the third-highest cause of death for young women aged 15–19) . . . these highly publicized and highly available cases lead people to ignore the data that suggest HIV can be contracted by sexual contact with anyone who has not been fully abstinent, has taken intravenous drugs, or has had sexual contact with a drug user, etc. Instead, people are likely to conclude once again that the risk to them is minimal. (p. 297)

What's more, although students know that condom use helps prevent HIV, they frequently engage in unprotected sex. Sexually active college students report that they used condoms less than 50% of the time when they had sex over the past year (Thompson et al., 1996). Many students involved in sexual relationships assume they are safe because they are monogamous: They know their partners and trust them. But as Suzanne Thompson and her colleagues report:

> The majority of college students in serious relationships are not monogamous, but rather serially monogamous. That is, they are having sex with only one partner at a time, but one monogamous relationship is followed by another. . . . One recent study of college women found that 95% described their romantic relationship as monogamous, yet as many as 41% reported having sex with someone other than their current partner the last time they engaged in intercourse. (p. 205)

BOX 2.1

SAFER SEX SNAPSHOT

What do young people really think about safer sex? What is their view of condoms and sex in the age of AIDS? This interview by Mark Fritz is with a 25-year-old heterosexual male from the Cleveland area. (*I* refers to interviewer, *R* to respondent.)

I: Are you sexually active?

R: Yes I am.

I: Have you demanded the use of condoms with your sexual partner?

R: I will wear a condom when I either am having sex with a woman for the first time or when she asks me to wear one.

I: When was the last time you had sexual relations?

R: Wow! Good question [laughing]. I would say it's been a couple months.

I: How do you feel about condom use in general?

R: I think they are okay. Nothing I'd write home about, but respecting yourself and your partner sometimes requires a calling above and beyond.

I: How do you think your partner feels about condom use?

R: Most women I have been with have never even brought the subject up. That kinda surprised me a bit because I figure they don't want to get pregnant. Then a friend of mine told me that by them not mentioning it tells you that they are on the pill. Though I'm not sure of the logic in that, when I think back it does seem pretty practical.

I: Why do you use condoms?

R: Ya know, I use condoms so that I don't get a girl pregnant. That is not what I want to do at this point in my life. They can be tricky about that.

I: Do you carry condoms with you when you go out?

R: I have one in my wallet all the time. At least over the past couple of months.

I: How do you personally get condoms?

R: Drug Mart, I guess. Any place that sells bathroom stuff will sell rubbers.

COMMENT: This man exhibits considerable respect for himself and female partners by insisting on condom use. However, he also says that women don't bring up the condom topic because they are on the pill. There is no evidence to support this view, and it is more a rationalization than a fact. What's more, even if women are on the pill, using birth control pills will not protect them from HIV infection.

But wait a minute. The overwhelming number of AIDS cases in the United States are found among gay men and injecting drug users. "Heterosexual AIDS in North America and Europe is, and will remain, rare," Robert Root-Bernstein (1993) notes, observing that "the chances that a healthy, drug-free heterosexual will contract AIDS from another heterosexual are so small they are hardly worth worrying about" (pp. 312–313). Experts across the scientific and political spectrums agree with this analysis.

And yet, bad things do happen to innocent people: Healthy individuals get cancer or contract viruses never before heard of (the odds of this happening are one in a million, but I bet you can think of someone you know personally who suddenly got very sick or died young). Although middle-class, heterosexual American high school and college students are not primarily at risk for HIV infection, handfuls of young people from these backgrounds will fall prey to HIV in the coming years. Sexually transmitted diseases like chlamydia and herpes are spreading at alarming rates, particularly among adolescents (Stolberg, 1998a). STDs produce lesions, which offer the HIV convenient access to an individual's bloodstream (Rushing, 1995). Although sexually transmitted infections don't cause HIV infection, they can increase the odds that a person will contract the AIDS virus.

Gay Men and Invulnerability.   It's troubling that gay men—who, as a group, are at considerable risk to get HIV/AIDS—also harbor illusions of invulnerability. Laurie Bauman and Karolynn Siegel (1987) asked 160 gay men to tell them how many times and with how many different sexual partners they participated in a variety of sexual activities during a 30-day period. The researchers grouped the practices into three categories: safe practices (hugging, kissing, mutual masturbation), low-risk activities (respondent inserts penis into partner's anus while using a condom), and risky practices (respondent inserts penis into partner's anus without using a condom). They also asked the men to rate the riskiness of their current sexual practices.

Sixty-six (41%) of the 160 men reported engaging in risky sexual practices. What's more, 55 (83%) of these 66 men perceived that these activities were of relatively low risk.

Although this study was conducted more than a decade ago, its conclusions still apply today. Gay men continue to unrealistically appraise the riskiness of their behavior (Altman, 1999b; Thompson et al., 1999). Rotello (1997) offers two reasons for this:

1. Unsafe sex is not followed by the swift and sure penalty of infection . . . [F]or each individual, the immediate risk of one unsafe encounter—the one they are about to have right now—often seems quite low and escapable, and statistically speaking they're right.

2. Even when infection does occur, illness is postponed for many years, per-

haps even decades... A 20-year-old gay man having unsafe sex today can quite logically assume that if he does get infected, he probably won't get sick until he reaches his 30s or, with today's improved drug therapies, even later. To many 20-year-olds, the age of 35 seems like a lifetime away. (p. 240)

It is ironic that the success of the new drugs in preventing death from AIDS has had an effect opposite to that which many expected: It has encouraged men to take new risks. Conceivably, sexually active gay men may be even more apt to assume they are invulnerable today than 10 to 15 years ago, when HIV infection could not be treated with drugs and almost invariably led to a quick and painful death. There are now new drugs—called protease inhibitors—that can help HIV-positive individuals survive the virus, in some cases for many years. Unfortunately, the drugs do not exert the same therapeutic effects on all men infected with HIV. "AIDS drugs don't work for everyone and aren't a cure for anyone," one AIDS prevention advocate said (Sternberg, 1999b, p. A1). Yet many gay men believe the drug therapies are cures or incorrectly assume that because the virus cannot be detected in their bloodstream they cannot transmit HIV (Altman, 1999b). Emboldened by these beliefs (rooted as they are in illusions of invulnerability), many men are returning to the unsafe sex fold and engaging in risky sexual practices. Indeed, one study found that the more optimistic men were about HIV drug treatments, the less inclined they were to use condoms during anal sex or to abstain from anal intercourse entirely (Altman, 1999b).

Thus, Bauman and Siegel's conclusions about risk distortion and denial among gay men hold true today. As the investigators perceptively observed in their original paper:

> When the AIDS epidemic occurred, certain sexual practices of gay men were suddenly defined as dangerous (i.e., potentially life threatening). To acknowledge and confront the fact that their past and present behavior put them at risk for AIDS may have been too threatening for many men. Some, therefore, tended to misperceive or distort the available public health information in ways that permitted them to appraise their behavior as less risky than it actually is. . . . However, denial is not always functional. While it successfully reduces emotional distress, it tends to interfere with taking direct action, which may be necessary in certain situations to optimize other goals such as safety and survival. (1987, pp. 346, 333)

BALANCE SHEET

Cognitive decision theories tell us a great deal about AIDS prevention behavior. They shed light on the reasons people do or don't take precautions against HIV infection. They illuminate the cognitive underpinnings of safer sex attitudes, help us predict behavior, and suggest AIDS communication campaign strategies that would not occur to most of us on our own.

Of the two models discussed in this chapter, the theory of reasoned action is more helpful because it takes into account people's need to go along with important others, spells out some of the factors that intervene between thought and action, and recognizes that a variable cannot influence behavior unless it is salient or occurs spontaneously to the individual. Perhaps most importantly, the TRA works: Condom attitudes, subjective norms, and intentions to use condoms are highly correlated with condom usage (Sheeran, Abraham, & Orbell, 1999).

Yet one bugaboo remains. Cognitive decision models—particularly the TRA—focus on intentions, but in the volatile arena of sex, intentions do not always predict behavior. Emotions and sexual arousal may overtake the best of intentions. Furthermore, safer sex differs from other behaviors that have been successfully forecast by the TRA in that "condom use depends on the availability of resources (e.g., a condom), opportunity (e.g., a prospective sexual partner), and interpersonal cooperation" (Sheeran et al., 1999, p. 121).

In many walks of life, intention to perform an action predicts behavior with great precision. In fact, for many people, intention to take an HIV test or to use condoms predicts behavior. But there are others for whom AIDS preventive intentions do not forecast behavior. A young heterosexual or gay man may know all about AIDS, even perceive he is vulnerable, and actually intend to engage in safe sex. But if our young lover is drunk or hooked on drugs, cognition is thrown out the window. He may succumb to other forces, such as emotion, the heated sexuality of the moment, or the desire to placate a partner (whom he originally planned to persuade to use a condom). The theory of reasoned action recognizes this problem more than do other approaches. Nonetheless, the theory has trouble explaining why some people who intend to use a condom succeed in practicing safer sex, while others with favorable intentions fail to translate intentions into behavior (Sheeran et al., 1999).

CONCLUSION

In this chapter, I argued that theory helps us better understand AIDS preventive behavior. I focused on two theories that loosely fall under the cognitive decision rubric. The theory of reasoned action asserts that attitude toward a behavior and subjective norm predict intention to engage in AIDS precautionary behaviors. The TRA pinpoints reasons why heterosexual young people, gay men, and injecting drug users don't always perform AIDS preventive behaviors.

The health belief model assumes that people are motivated to take cognitive steps to protect themselves against disease. Four key factors—perceived severity, perceived susceptibility, perceived benefits, and perceived barriers—influence health-related behavior. By explicating and studying these cognitions, the HBM has helped researchers and practitioners better understand why people don't always follow medical advice.

One of the bugaboos of the HBM is the illusion of invulnerability, or people's reluctance to acknowledge that they are personally vulnerable to negative outcomes, like HIV infection. We assume invulnerability because it increases our sense of personal control and jibes with our stereotypes of those most susceptible to disease. Teenagers and college students are especially prone to minimize their susceptibility to AIDS.

Critics have noted that the HBM and TRA are not ideally suited to predicting sexual behavior because emotional and physiological factors can inhibit the translation of thoughts into action. Although this is a fair criticism, the fact remains that variables emphasized by the theories—the TRA in particular—predict behavior rather handsomely. And while diverse psychological, communication, and cultural factors must be considered if we are to predict AIDS prevention behavior, there is no question that cognitive decision models have advanced knowledge of the psychology of HIV infection.

CHAPTER THREE

Social Psychological and Communication Perspectives on Unsafe Sex

Mark Ebenhoch is talking with a reporter about the strange, circuitous path that took him from the Marines to HIV infection. He "has on his 'command' voice: the voice of fearless authority he learned during 12 years in the Marines," reporter Jesse Green (1996) tells us. However, as Green relates:

A fearless voice hardly seems appropriate now, in my hotel room, talking about sex; he [Ebenhoch] wants to get rid of it, but it keeps re-emerging . . . So he talks about what has brought him to this state—he is HIV negative but wonders how long he can hold on—as if he were announcing a baseball game. "Heck, I'd been such a good boy, followed my church upbringing, wouldn't cuss, even in the corps. I was celibate for 13 years instead of being gay! So then, last year when I finally came out, I came out flying like a bat out of hell. Wednesday, Friday, Saturday I'd go to this bar called Friends, which was outside a military base that was notorious for gay bashings. I'd walk in and it was a really friendly atmosphere, so I sat down and ordered a beer. Once, this guy, not even my type really, sat down next to me. He was military, which I could tell from his haircut, and it didn't take that long, a drink or two and a couple cigarettes, before he said, 'Do you want to go do something?' And it was like, O.K., let's go . . .

"In California the bars give you the condoms free; not in North Carolina, where I was living then. And no one brings it up. It's not thought about. Well, for a split second, but I say to myself: I know this is a marine, I know he gets checked every six months and he's probably the safest bet in the world. And this one was married.

"It was like I was finally inside the candy store I'd been looking at forever. I wasn't about to deny myself now. So during that time, those two or three months, I guess I had over 20 partners. A lot of the time I was drunk, though, so I can't say for sure. Sometimes you'd go home with somebody you might not really want because of loneliness, and in that position I sure wouldn't mention safe sex. I'd always wait for them to say something about it." He nods his head sharply, as if dismissing an underling. "But no one did. . . ."

Mark Ebenhoch's command voice, which hasn't worked any better for him than it has for AIDS educators, is almost completely gone now. Even over the phone, when I speak to him in mid-July, I can hear the change. His affair with B. has ended unhappily and, he adds, almost as an afterthought, he has some news we have both been fearing: he is finally HIV-positive himself. A psychiatrist has put him on antidepressants. "Sometimes I think that if I had gotten help three years ago—emotional help, psychiatric help—I most likely wouldn't be positive now. I'd have had a clearer head. But really, it was my own fault. There's no other way around it." (pp. 39–40, 85)

Sadly, Mark Ebenhoch is one of many gay men who engage in unsafe sex, despite knowing better. To be sure, sizable numbers of gay men remain free of infection, continuing to subscribe to what Rotello (1997) calls "the condom code" (see also Bolton, 1992; Ekstrand & Coates, 1990; Rogers et al., 1995). But not all men regularly take precautions against risky sex. Some of those who practiced safer sex seem to have relapsed into unsafe sexual behavior and scores of younger gay men, convinced of their immortality, routinely engage in unprotected sexual intercourse (Kalichman, Kelly, & Rompa, 1997; Rotello, 1997). Some of these men have contracted the AIDS virus. In a similar fashion, other at-risk individuals—heterosexuals with many sex partners, injecting drug users, and poor women of color—regularly engage in sexual practices that put them at risk to contract HIV/AIDS.

In the absence of an AIDS vaccine, education remains a major weapon in the battle against HIV infection. Yet to educate—or, more precisely, persuade—people to take precautions against AIDS, an understanding of the dynamics of their safer sex attitudes and behaviors is needed. Campaign practitioners cannot influence people unless they understand the mental goblins and cognitive traps that impede people's efforts to change. Strangely enough, this brings us back to theory. As noted in chapter 2, theory and research shed light on attitudes and suggest strategies for attitude change. This chapter continues the explication of social scientific theories of AIDS risk reduction, focusing on social psychological and interpersonal communication perspectives.

THEORY OF PLANNED BEHAVIOR

Icek Ajzen (1991), who helped develop the Theory of Reasoned Action, observed that the TRA is useful in predicting behaviors over which people have volitional control, but is less helpful in explaining actions that are not under people's control. Ajzen argues that when people perceive that they can't control a particular behavior, they are less capable of translating intention into action. Under these circumstances, adding perceived behavioral control to the TRA mix of attitude, subjective norm, and intention should increase accuracy of behavioral prediction.

Safer sex would seem to be one of those behaviors over which people do not always have volitional control. Successful performance of the behavior requires the availability of a condom and cooperation between sex partners, neither of which is always under an individual's control. Furthermore, as Meg Gerrard, Frederick Gibbons, and Brad Bushman (1996) observed:

> The unique nature of the sex drive contributes to the fact that decisions about sex are oftentimes made in the heat of the moment—when the person is emotionally and physically aroused—rather than after careful, or even rational, deliberation . . . The literature suggests that decisions regarding sexual risk taking are highly vulnerable to emotional interference and, therefore, may not be as rational as decisions involving precautionary behaviors that are less emotion-laden, such as wearing a seat belt or getting a flu shot. (pp. 400–401)

There are other reasons why people may perceive that they have little control over safer sex. Some young heterosexuals, concerned that their partner will get angry if they suggest using a condom, believe there is little they can do to facilitate cooperation. Injecting drug users, knowing that drugs reduce cognitive functioning, may fear that they can't "get it together" to use a condom during the heat of the moment. Gay men who suffer from abnormal sexual compulsion may be psychologically unable to control their urge for unsafe sex (e.g., Kalichman, Greenberg, & Abel, 1997). Male prostitutes, who must comply with their clients' sexual needs, believe that the client controls the sexual encounter (Joffe & Dockrell, 1995). Women, particularly those living in impoverished conditions, frequently fear that attempts to exert control over safer sex communication will doom a relationship or result in their being physically assaulted (Amaro, 1995).

Believing that safer sexual behaviors are beyond their control, such individuals may not always be capable of translating attitudes into intentions or intentions into behavior. The theory of planned behavior helps us remedy this problem. Researchers assess perceptions of behavioral control and determine whether inclusion of perceived behavioral control increases ability to predict safer sex behavior. Perceived behavioral control over condom use has been assessed by questions like these:

How difficult is it for you to use condoms with new sexual partners?

1   2   3   4   5   6   7

Very Difficult   Not At All Difficult

Now this is just a "what if" question, but if you wanted to use a condom every time you have vaginal sex with your main partner, how sure are you that you could?

1   2   3   4   5   6   7

Extremely Sure I Could Not   Extremely Sure I Could

(Reinecke, Schmidt, & Ajzen, 1996, p. 755; Corby, Jamner, & Wolitski, 1996, p. 60)

Research shows that the more control people believe they have over condom use, the more likely they are to intend to use condoms, and to translate intentions into condom use behavior (Corby et al., 1996; Reinecke et al., 1996). Conversely, the lower people's perceived control over condom use, the less likely they are to translate safer sex intentions into action. Campaign practitioners must develop creative ways to teach people that they can control the use and discussion of condoms in intimate sexual settings.

SOCIAL COGNITIVE THEORY

Social cognitive theory puts a premium on *self-efficacy*, the belief that one can influence things that happen in everyday life. More specifically, perceived self-efficacy is an individual's conviction that he or she can successfully perform behaviors necessary to produce desired outcomes (Bandura, 1977, 1992). Social cognitive theory assumes that people learn they can influence events (or that they can't) through observation of role models, verbal persuasion, success and failure experiences, and interpretation of these outcomes. The theory's architect, Albert Bandura (1998), notes:

> Among the mechanisms of human agency, none is more central, or pervasive than beliefs of personal efficacy. It is the foundation of human agency. Unless people believe they can produce desired effects by their actions, they have little incentive to act or to persevere in the face of difficulties. . . . Human well-being and accomplishments require an optimistic and resilient efficacy. This is because the normative daily realities are strewn with difficulties. They are full of frustrations, impediments, adversities, failures, setbacks, conflicts, and inequities. It requires a resilient sense of efficacy to override such dissuading conditions. (p. 2)

Social cognitive theory places considerable emphasis on confidence—believing one can master difficult tasks. According to the theory, people who have a strong sense of personal efficacy take on difficult tasks, become involved in challenging activities, recover from defeat, and persist in the face of failure. Those who have a low sense of efficacy are more apt to avoid challenging tasks, focus on personal shortcomings rather than how to master daunting situations, and surrender quickly in the face of failure (Bandura, 1995).

Applied to HIV prevention, social cognitive theory suggests that the more efficacious people feel about talking to partners about safer sex, or exerting control over sexual activities, the more likely they are to undertake the challenge of bringing up the subject of safer sex, persist in the face of partner objections, and translate safer sex intentions into behavior. By contrast, those with low perceived self-efficacy may yield when a partner resists their appeal to use a condom, become depressed after unsuccessful attempts to negotiate condom use, and fail to practice safer sex even if they harbor positive intentions.

Thus far I have used the term *self-efficacy* but have not described how it is assessed in social psychological surveys. Leave it to researchers to devise a questionnaire to measure the concept! Linda Brafford and Kenneth Beck (1991) developed a professional, reliable, and valid condom use self-efficacy scale. See if you *strongly agree, agree,* are *undecided, disagree,* or *strongly disagree* with these statements:

1. I feel confident I could purchase condoms without feeling embarrassed.
2. I would feel comfortable discussing condom use with a potential sexual partner before we ever engaged in intercourse.
3. If I were to suggest using a condom to a partner, I would feel afraid that he or she would reject me.
4. I would not feel confident suggesting using condoms with a new partner because I would be afraid he or she would think I thought they had a sexually transmitted disease.
5. I feel confident that I would remember to use a condom even after I have been drinking.
6. I would feel embarrassed to put a condom on myself or my partner.
7. I feel confident I could stop to put a condom on myself or my partner even in the heat of passion. (p. 221; see also Brien et al., 1994)

Research shows that the more people respond efficaciously to questions like these—that is, the higher their perceived self-efficacy about using condoms—the more likely they are to engage in AIDS preventive behaviors, like safer sex (Bakker, Buunk, & Manstead, 1997; Basen-Engquist, 1992; Carvajal, Garner, & Evans, 1998; Goldman & Harlow, 1993; Marin et al., 1998; McKusick et al., 1990; Smith et al., 1996; Wulfert, Wan, & Backus, 1996). Yet self-efficacy is not a static entity. Those with low perceived self-efficacy regarding safer sex can change their beliefs if they are motivated to do so and receive compelling information from credible sources. Bandura argues that communication campaigns can increase self-efficacy by doing several things. In particular, campaigns should strive to: (a) impart accurate information to increase awareness of health risks, (b) teach social and self-management skills through modeling, (c) offer extensive practice in these skills to increase the odds that people will perform them in real life situations, and (d) provide social support to maintain behavioral change.

Although the concept of self-efficacy has a certain ambiguity (Kirsch, 1995), the theory that incorporates it has important strengths. It offers specific insights into why people do not always engage in AIDS precautionary behaviors and suggests strategies for persuasion campaigns, as I show in chapter 5.

INTERPERSONAL COMMUNICATION

Talking about safer sex should be easy.

It doesn't require an advanced degree to bring up the topic. Most people know what they are supposed to say and why saying it is so important. Yet research documents that young people are notoriously reluctant to discuss safer sex with their romantic partners (Bowen & Michal-Johnson, 1989; Cline, Johnson, & Freeman, 1992). It turns out that communicating about these issues is no simple matter. Talking about AIDS is an emotional volcano, seemingly as threatening to the vulnerable self-concept as HIV is to the human body.

In exploring the dynamics of sexual communication, I call on research that transcends the individual and focuses instead on communication between people—on ways people negotiate safer sex, devise strategies to obtain interpersonal goals, and jointly construct sexual encounters. Communication about safer sex frequently involves condom use, but it is not limited to this topic. It can also include broader discussions of a partner's sexual values, HIV testing, the possibility of getting tested together, and even agreeing to practice safer sex with other people if both partners choose not to be monogamous (Kalichman, 1998).

AIDS Communication Between Heterosexual College Students

Public health pamphlets urge people to talk frankly about safer sex with their partners. More than a decade ago, the Surgeon General's (1988) message to the public on AIDS warned that "If you know someone well enough to have sex, then you should be able to talk about AIDS. If someone is unwilling to talk, you shouldn't have sex" (p. 4). Communication scholars echo this advice, noting that "talk can be a primary vehicle for personalizing AIDS risk, convincing the partner to use preventive measures (e.g., condoms) and helping partners decide on mutually acceptable, and safe, sexual practices" (Waldron, Caughlin, & Jackson, 1995, p. 250).

So what's the scoop? Are people talking about AIDS or sexual protection? Most of the research on college students' communication about safer sex was conducted several years back, so caution needs to be exercised in interpreting the results. Norms have loosened and safer sex is a more acceptable topic to discuss than it was in the early 1990s. Nonetheless, the available research offers insights into young people's communication about these issues.

Students do talk with sexual partners about AIDS—nearly two thirds of a university sample said they discussed this topic with romantic partners (Cline et al., 1992). Yet such conversations often don't touch on sensitive issues, like fears and attitudes about AIDS (Bowen & Michal-Johnson, 1989). Rebecca Cline and her colleagues (1992) found that only one in five sexually experienced respondents reported discussing safer sex with partners. Of these, only one third talked about condom use. "The upshot is that only 6.3% of the sexually experienced sample reporting having AIDS-related discussions that focused on efficacious means of AIDS prevention," Cline concluded (p. 53).

Why don't young people talk openly about condom use? "Most people are aware that they should be talking about these issues," Sheryl Perlmutter Bowen and Paula Michal-Johnson (1989) note, "but for many reasons they choose not to do so" (p. 12). Safer sex appears to be an off-limits subject in many romantic relationships. Consider that there are a number of taboo topics in close relationships, including the state of the relationship, extrarelationship activity, relationship norms, prior relationships, conflict-generating topics, and self-disclosures perceived as unpleasant to discuss (Baxter & Wilmot, 1985). Condom use touches on all of these.

If a relationship partner brings up the subject of condoms, he or she runs the risk of the other person suspecting that she or he has HIV or an STD. Broaching the topic may also insult the other party. As one student put it, "It's like you're saying, 'I think you've slept around'" (Hammer et al., 1996, p. 387). Mentioning condoms can also destroy the mood. One male respondent in a University of Connecticut study illustrated the problem by poking fun at the interruption to reach for a condom: "Excuse me, I have to put on my Trojan" (Hammer et al., 1996, p. 383). For other students, condoms bring to mind a number of negative images (AIDS, death, homosexuality) that both parties would rather avoid. This is not to say that no one broaches the issue. Some do. But many don't, fearing that a discussion might harm a blossoming relationship. As Timothy Edgar and his colleagues (1992) observed, "heterosexual college students do have uncertainties about new sexual partners, but the motivation to reduce these uncertainties is driven more by concern about the potential for developing the relationship than by anxiety about AIDS or other STDs" (p. 100).

Such concern does make sense. "Relationship partners provide intimacy and a source of commitment," Jill Hammer and her colleagues (1996, p. 376) remind us. Being involved in a relationship—particularly a loving one—gives young people enormous joy, satisfaction, self-esteem rewards and, perhaps most of all, helps reduce the pain of loneliness. Who would want to risk it all by mentioning HIV, particularly when students believe that their risk of contracting the virus is infinitesimally small? Moreover, couples frequently begin having sex before they are comfortable talking about intimate emotional issues. Cultural norms and gender inequality also inhibit honest discussion of safer sex (see chapter 4).

One factor that has an especially strong impact on condom communication is the phase of the romantic relationship. Some college students talk more about condom use in casual sexual relationships—one night stands. Condom use is more likely to occur in casual than serious sexual relationships (Hammer et al., 1996; Kalichman, 1998; Reisen & Poppen, 1995). Once a relationship gets serious, condom use seems to drop off—and perhaps so too does communication about safer sex. Young people incorrectly believe that a monogamous relationship is safe and are concerned that initiating safer-sex behaviors might threaten trust or intimacy. One student in the University of Connecticut study claimed that continuing to use condoms in a steady relationship "almost *proves* . . . a lack of trust" (Hammer et al., 1996, p. 385). For many college students, the cost of using condoms in a long-term relationship exceeds the benefits of AIDS prevention. Yet as Hammer and her associates point out, "although relationship members tend to see each other through rose-colored glasses, somehow we need to convey the message, as stated by a participant, that 'you can trust someone with your heart and still not trust them with your life'" (p. 393).

Interpersonal Communication Dynamics

You know how delicate and dynamic communication about sex can be. You know how tricky it can be to bring up sensitive topics, like what you want a lover to do during sex, what you don't like, and what to do about sexual protection. "Sex may be one of life's greatest pleasures," Sandra Metts and Brian Spitzberg (1996) note, "but it is also a source of some of our thorniest interpersonal and social problems" (p. 49).

Interpersonal communication scholars view sexual communication as a complex, dynamic process, in which "sexual partners are *active participants,* who each have their own set of *goals* and the ability to choose *strategies* to maximize goal achievement" (Miller et al., 1993, p. 87). Furthermore, people have diverse, sometimes conflicting goals during sex—fulfilling sexual desire, maintaining a positive self-image, pleasing their partner, strengthening the relationship, relieving tension, and preserving health. Three interpersonal and intrapersonal processes are particularly important: **scripts, plans, and compliance-gaining.**

Scripts. A *script* approach views people as sexual actors who have learned the cultural rules—the societal stageplay—for what people do when they want to initiate and consummate sexual activity. Sexual scripts are "cognitive structures specifying appropriate goals in sexually relevant contexts and specifying sequences of behavior . . . that are appropriate and efficacious for achieving those goals" (Metts & Spitzberg, 1996, p. 50). Scripts vary as a function of the culture and gender orientation of sexual partners. The traditional script for heterosexual behavior is for men to initiate action and evade limits on sexual activity; women are expected to be more passive and to place limits on sex (Edgar & Fitzpatrick, 1993). Among gay men, the script for sex in one context—the bathhouse—is that the man "on top" makes decisions about condom usage (Elwood & Williams, 1999, p. 126). The man on the bottom—the receptive partner—is the subservient individual, who is expected to show respect by remaining silent, even if he wants to initiate condom use.

People use scripts to plot out appropriate activities during sex (Edgar & Fitzpatrick, 1993). Individuals may depart from the script but are aware of the expected sequences of sexual behavior in a dating or love-making situation (see Fig. 3.1). In many cases, people follow scripts automatically, without much conscious deliberation or systematic thinking.

There are two phases in the use of sexual scripts: (a) information-seeking and (b) requesting or not requesting condom use (Metts & Fitzpatrick, 1992). During the first phase, individuals can passively gather information about partner

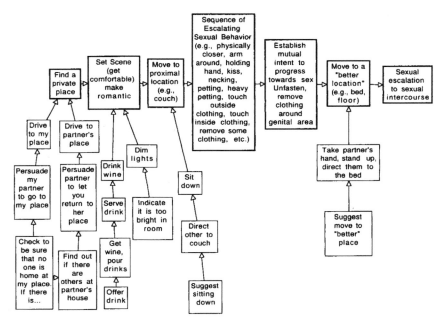

FIG. 3.1.   Standard initiator sexual script for a "one-night stand." From "Negotiating safe sex: Interpersonal dynamics" (p. 98), by L. C. Miller, B. A. Bettencourt, S. C. De Bro, and V. Hoffman. In J. B. Pryor and G. D. Reeder (Eds.), *The Social Psychology of HIV Infection,* 1993, Hillsdale, NJ: Lawrence Erlbaum Associates.

riskiness, as many college students do when they assess risk through physical appearance. As one female student at Berkeley put it, "you look for signs, blisters, physical manifestations. But if someone doesn't look as if they have a disease, you don't use a condom" (Edgar, Freimuth, & Hammond, 1988, p. 62). Other students gather information passively by relying on simple rules like "if you just met them, you use a condom . . . if it's long term, you aren't going to worry" (Williams et al., 1992, pp. 926–927). Needless to say, both these information strategies are flawed because people can be infected with HIV yet not exhibit physical signs, and long-term partners can have contracted the virus but either not know or not tell sex partners.

Bringing up the condom topic can sometimes be so scary that young people dance around it, asking questions about the individual's riskiness in ways that guarantee they will get the answer they want—for example,"You don't have AIDS, do you? I didn't think so"; conversation ceases and petting begins (Snyder & Swann, 1978).

During the second phase of script use, individuals can express a desire to use a condom or request the partner use a condom. Numerous factors influence this communicative decision, including perceptions of how the request will be seen by the other and the degree to which it is consistent with cultural norms.

Is condom use a component of contemporary sexual scripts? Has discussion of sexual protection become an accepted part of the sexual interaction sequence? While early studies of heterosexual college students found that condoms did not figure prominently in the casual sex scenario (Edgar & Fitzpatrick, 1993; Miller et al., 1993), later work indicates that safer sex is a part of young people's scripts. As Metts and Spitzberg (1996) note: "Many sexually active people have incorporated a condom use contingency into their larger sexual scripts. The association between condoms and responsible sex in public discourse seems to have provided a frame of legitimacy for the use of condoms" (p. 81).

As encouraging as these findings are, there is darker side to this research: Even though sexually active young people increasingly talk about condoms with partners, they do not always tell the truth about their previous sexual histories (Cochran & Mays, 1990; Mays & Cochran, 1993). What's more, despite increases in safer sexual communication, unprotected sex among heterosexual college students, as well as those at greater risk for HIV infection, continues apace (e.g., Overby & Kegeles, 1994).

Plans.   *Plans* are cognitive constructs that intervene between thought and action. They may be crucial concepts in the domain of safer sex. Many people may want to discuss condoms with their partners, but fail because they lack a plan for how to do so. The ministrations of the moment or desire to please a lover frequently overcome safer sex intentions.

The term *plan* has a very specific meaning in interpersonal communication research. According to Charles Berger (1988), a plan "specifies the actions that are necessary for the attainment of a goal or several goals" (p. 96). Unlike scripts, plans are strategically and consciously generated to achieve a particular goal. Plans vary in their complexity, specificity, and quality (Waldron, 1997). Situational factors influence the content of people's plans (Berger, 1997), and individuals differ in the effectiveness with which they use plans (Berger & Bell, 1988). In a study that applied plan theory to AIDS, Waldron and his colleagues (1995) found that communicators who produced a greater number of plans and those who developed more specific plans were better able to guide discussions of safer sex.

Compliance-Gaining.   Just how does one person persuade another to engage in safer sex? What strategies do people use to gain compliance? These questions are addressed in an area of interpersonal persuasion research known as compliance-gaining.

Compliance-gaining is defined as a "communicative behavior in which an agent engages so as to elicit from a target some agent-selected behavior" (Wheeless, Barraclough, & Stewart, 1983, p. 111). Researchers have explored the strategies individuals use to gain compliance in a variety of settings, employing a host of different techniques to understand how ordinary people attempt to persuade others to go along with their requests. While procedures to measure compliance-gaining have been criticized for lack of clarity, they nonetheless offer clues about how people attempt to secure agreement from others (Seibold, Cantrill, & Meyers, 1994).

Applying compliance-gaining models to safer sex is dicey because safer sex differs in three ways from other arenas in which people try to gain compliance. First, as Edgar (1992) observes:

> Unlike other behaviors for the protection of one's health, condom use is not a unilateral practice. Unless one partner is completely naive to the realities of sex, condoms cannot be used unobtrusively. Agreement and cooperation are necessary conditions for completion of the precautionary behavior. (p. 47)

Second, although people like to deny it, the consequences of noncompliance with a request for safer sex are more serious than in other domains. If a relational partner declines a lover's plaintive plea to get married, the result will be disappointment and hurt feelings, but not infection or death (Edgar & Fitzpatrick, 1988). Third, safer sex discussions touch on more sexual and intense emotional issues than do compliance-gaining requests in other contexts.

How do people try to influence a partner to use a condom? Sherrine De Bro and her colleagues (1994) explored this issue, asking heterosexual college students to indicate how they would try to persuade a date to use a condom. Six strategies emerged:

> *Reward:* "I would emphasize that (partner's) respect for my feelings about using a condom would really enhance our relationship."
>
> *Emotional coercion:* "I would let (partner) know that I would be upset and angry at (him or her) for not wanting to use a condom."
>
> *Risk information:* "I would tell (partner) that it's risky to have sex without a condom. We would both be safer from disease if we use a condom."
>
> *Deception:* "Even though I want to use a condom because I'm worried about sexually transmitted diseases, I'd make up a different reason to tell (him/her)."
>
> *Seduction:* "Before (partner) had a chance to object to the use of a condom, I would get (him/her) so 'turned on' that (he/she) would forget about the condom."
>
> *Withhold sex:* "I would just tell (partner) that I will make love only if we use a condom." (adapted from De Bro, Campbell, & Peplau, 1994, p. 171)

Female participants in De Bro's study viewed reward, emotional coercion, risk information, and withholding sex as more comfortable strategies than did male participants. Men, on the other hand, rated seduction as a more comfortable strategy than did women. Importantly, this was an exploratory study; we don't know the degree to which these strategies would be used in an actual sit-uations nor how effective they are.

Summary. Safer sex communication is a cauldron of competing goals, emo-tional agendas, and dynamic compliance-gaining strategies. Far from occurring in a vacuum, communication about condoms "occurs in a complex, value-laden, interpersonal context—one in which the participants are likely to be aroused both emotionally and physically and are faced with intense impression management concerns" (Bryan, Aiken, & West, 1999, p. 285).

Women are sometimes reluctant to propose condom use because they fear it will reduce their attractiveness or trigger angry responses from men. Men fear that broaching the condom topic will make them seem less "macho" in women's eyes or will give women the opportunity to reject their sexual ad-vances (Bryan et al., 1999). For many people, sexual scripts, uncertainty about how a partner will react to a compliance-gaining strategy, and maintaining inti-macy exert a stronger impact on decisions to talk about condoms than do health concerns emphasized by the Health Belief Model (Bryan, Aiken, & West, 1999; Kellar-Guenther, 1999).

Unfortunately, campaigns to increase safer sex talk rarely consider such fac-tors. They suggest only that people talk frankly about condom use. The lesson from interpersonal communication research is that campaigns will fail unless they take into account what researchers know about the emotional dynamics of sexual communication (see Boxes 3.1 and 3.2).

FUNCTIONAL THEORY PERSPECTIVE ON UNSAFE SEX

The models discussed so far in this chapter—planned behavior, social cogni-tion, and interpersonal communication—do not assume that AIDS prevention behavior is always rational or carefully planned out. But the theories do use a cognitive language to describe safer sex, and they assume that with increased skills training people can be taught to change unsafe sex behaviors. There is considerable merit to these approaches: at the same time, no theory can explain all aspects of a phenomenon, and (although they implicitly take emotions into account) these models do not adequately account for the irrationality of sex. In particular, the theories do not explain why so many people who know better continue to engage in unsafe sexual behaviors that could put their own or a partner's health in jeopardy. To understand the emotional dynamics of unsafe sex, I turn to functional theories of attitude (Katz, 1960; Snyder, 1987). Func-tional approaches assume that our attitudes and behaviors are not always ra-tional and that we hold attitudes because they perform functions, or allow us to satisfy powerful human needs.

Functional theory is particularly helpful in explaining a disturbing—and seemingly baffling—development: continued evidence of unsafe sex among gay

---

BOX 3.1

SAFER SEX SNAPSHOT

What do young people really think about safer sex? What is their view of condoms and sex in the age of AIDS? In this interview by Mark Fritz, a 19-year-old heterosexual woman who recently graduated from high school offers her opinions. (*I* refers to interviewer, *R* to respondent.)

I: Are you sexually active?

R: Well, yes.

I: Have you demanded the use of condoms with your sexual partner?

R: No. Don't get me wrong . . . it isn't like I sleep around or anything . . . it is just that I really don't have the heart to stop everything and ask my boyfriend to put on this rubber glove [laughing] and then try and get back in the mood.

I: When was the last time you had sexual relations?

R: My boyfriend and me did it about a week ago. I can't remember exactly when though.

I: How do you feel about condom use in general?

R: I don't want to get pregnant. I'm on the pill, but if my boyfriend can help me by wearing a condom then I would like that.

I: How do you think your partner feels about condom use?

R: Oh I know how guys feel about it [laughing]. All the arguments are the same. I feel sorry for them. My boyfriend, I mean, I want him to feel good when we are in bed. Since I am on the pill, I don't really mind if he doesn't use a rubber.

I: Why do you use condoms?

R: To not get pregnant. Right?

I: Do you carry condoms with you when you go out?

R: No, I don't. I suppose my boyfriend carries one in his wallet. Why? I don't know since he has me.

I: How do you personally get condoms?

R: [laughing] I went to buy some at Revco around from my apartment and the guy there I went to high school with. He is looking at me kinda weird and I am nervous. That is the last time I will ever buy rubbers anywhere near where I live now or where I used to live!

COMMENT: This woman is delightfully open about her sexual attitudes. However, like other young women, she is reluctant to talk her boyfriend into using a condom. She might benefit by gaining communication skills, such as those described in this chapter and chapter 5.

BOX 3.2

SAFER SEX SNAPSHOT

This final interview is with a 25-year-old gay student from the Cleveland area.

I: Are you sexually active?

R: Yes, very.

I: Have you demanded the use of condoms with your sexual partner?

R: I don't have a regular partner. I party a lot though and will ask my partners to use a condom as I will.

I: When was the last time you had sexual relations?

R: Do I really have to answer that? I don't want to answer that.

I: How do you feel about condom use in general?

R: I think that they are essential in helping stop the spread of AIDS. In the gay community, as you are aware, there is a real need to protect ourselves from killing each other off.

I: How do you think your partner feels about condom use?

R: Most of them prefer to be safe and use a condom. However, there are others that really don't want to use them. I try to stay away from those people because they are just tempting fate.

I: Why do you use condoms?

R: Unless they come up with something better, I prefer to have a little less sensation and a whole lot more of life to live. On the whole, it balances out.

I: Do you carry condoms with you when you go out?

R: I always carry more than one with me when I go out.

I: How do you personally get condoms?

R: You're joking, right? I get them at the drugstore. Where else does one go to buy rubbers? K-Mart?

I: How many times do you use a single condom?

I: I know the answer is once, but I actually know some people that have had sex with someone and used the condom more than once, they were so excited!

R: Do you think about AIDS much?

I: AIDS is something I think about all the time. It has to be. My lifestyle dictates that I am aware and very cautious. I know that. I know that society isn't supportive of what I do and how I choose to live, but it is my life. Shit, I don't want to die and I certainly don't want to die the way some of my friends have died. I am 25 and I shouldn't be experiencing the deaths of so many of my friends as I have. This is something that should happen to you when you are in your 60s, not your 20s. You know, I have lost 12 friends in

(Box continues)

BOX 3.2 (Continued)

the last 7 years. [He starts to tear up]. I don't have a strong personality that I can just blow away what I feel. These were some of my closest friends. I don't know . . . I don't know.

COMMENT. This young man is mature enough to realize the dangers of unsafe sex, and he is committed to using condoms. It is disturbing that some of his friends apparently used the same condom more than once. The man's last comment poignantly reminds us of the toll AIDS has taken among the young.

---

men, many of whom are highly aware of the dangers of unsafe sex and have even taught others to use appropriate cautions (Rotello, 1997). Consider the following statistics:

• Forty-three percent of a sample of 99 gay men from three West Coast cities reported engaging in unprotected anal sexual intercourse over the previous 6 months (Hays, Kegeles, & Coates, 1990).

• A study of Puerto Rican men in New York City found that condoms were employed inconsistently or not at all by half of the men who reported having anal sex with other men. Forty-one percent of the men were HIV-positive or assumed they were positive (Carballo-Diéguez & Dolezal, 1996).

• Thirty-nine percent of a cohort of HIV-positive gay and bisexual men from a Midwestern city reported engaging in unprotected anal intercourse over the previous 3 months. Sixty-seven percent of these men participated in anal sex with two or more partners, sometimes under the influence of drugs (Kalichman et al., 1997).

• In a study of 75 committed gay male couples of opposite HIV status (HIV-positive and HIV-negative), researchers found that in 50 (67%) of the couples, one or both partners reported having participated in sex outside the relationship. Some 25% of the men reported engaging in unprotected anal sex during one-night stands. Note that some of those who did not use condoms were HIV-positive (Wagner, Remien, & Carballo-Diéguez, 1998).

How can we explain these findings? Functional theory suggests that the reason gay men engage in such wildly unsafe sexual behavior is that sex satisfies important psychological needs. I discuss several of these needs, calling on theory and anecdotal accounts.

1. *Sexual validation.* Writer and gay activist Michelangelo Signorile (1997) observes that "a greater percentage of gay men than straight men are highly concerned with their physical appearance" (p. 10). Many of these guys work out with weights regularly, are consumed with achieving a masculine ideal, and

focus endlessly on sex. As Jeremy, a gay lawyer from Washington, DC, told Signorile, "There's nothing that can make me feel better if I'm feeling down than getting laid" (p. 20). For men like Jeremy, risky sexual behaviors are physically and emotionally satisfying. They provide excitement, adventure, and novelty (Ames, Atchinson, & Rose, 1995; Gold & Skinner, 1992; Kalichman, Heckman, & Kelly, 1996). Sexual adventure keeps some men going.

2. *Emotional intimacy.* Gay men, like their heterosexual counterparts, practice unsafe sex because it provides emotional commitment. As one man told researchers Joseph P. Stokes and John L. Peterson (1998), "I may [have sex] out of loneliness. I just need the companionship." Said another, "We all want to be accepted; we want to be loved; we want to be understood . . . , which is why we have a lot of sexual partners a lot of times." A third remarked that "I was so in love with this young man and so desperate to be loved and have a sense of belonging that I was willing to forego the condom just to gain this man's love and acceptance . . . I was willing to contract this deadly disease just to prove my love to this young man or just to have him—for us to become one" (p. 288).

3. *Compensating for feeling of inferiority.* During childhood, many gay men come to recognize that it is hard for them to bond or fit in with other guys. "That difference," Signorile observed, "often keeps them excluded from the typical kind of macho, heterosexual teenage camaraderie and bonding" (p. 138). Once they begin hanging out in the gay sexual world, these men vow never to be left out by the in crowd, which in their minds consists of super-attractive, highly sexualized gay men. One man told Stokes and Peterson that if he has low self-esteem, he wants a sexual experience "at any cost. I would do whatever it takes to ensure that I continue to have a sexual experience" (p. 288).

4. *Escape from stress.* Contrary to cognitive decision models, people do not always act in their rational self-interest. Some men, like Dostoevsky's (1960) underground man, relish behaving spontaneously, in ways that defy rational analysis. Harboring positive attitudes toward unsafe sex and purposefully engaging in it would seem to be inexplicable or incomprehensible until one recognizes that some behavior is motivated by a need for escape (McKirnan, Ostrow, & Hope, 1996).

Gay men face extraordinary pressure, resulting from both society's prejudices and the realization that the cost of a fulfilling sexual relationship may be HIV infection. Ironically, unbridled sex can take men's minds off these issues. Unsafe sex can become a powerful reinforcer, as D. J. McKirnan and his colleagues (1996) note, applying cognitive learning theory to homosexual sex:

> For a given individual, sexuality may become associated with physical settings such as bars, clubs, baths, or "cruise" areas, certain partners, or ancillary behaviors such as substance use. These stimuli may come to elicit not only sexual arousal, but the anxiety, negative affect, and aversive cognitive restraint that accompany awareness of HIV risk. If the person learns to be cognitively disengaged

in response to the stimulus—by enacting a relatively "mindless" sexual script, and/or using alcohol or drugs—he receives powerful rewards both from sexual satisfaction, and from the lowering of anxiety over HIV. (p. 662)

In other words, unsafe sex provides an escape from HIV risk, making life exciting and desirable. It is important to emphasize that not all gay men engage in unprotected sex. Many enjoy a monogamous relationship with a partner and avoid unsafe sexual experiences. However, some do engage in risky sexual practices that endanger not only their health but that of their partners. One can lament that these men participate in risky sex and criticize the ethics of HIV-positive men who put their partners at risk for infection. This is the subject for another discussion. The task of this book is to understand AIDS prevention attitudes and to suggest theory-based strategies to change them. In most instances, the best way to change behavior is not to moralize about it but to understand things from the individual's perspective and help the person make needed changes. Functional theory helps to do this.

CONCLUSION

In this chapter I have discussed theories that do not assume a totally rational model of AIDS prevention behavior. The theory of planned behavior stipulates that people do not always have control over their ability to engage in safer sex. The theory argues that condom use can be predicted more accurately by considering perceived control over condom use, in addition to attitude, subjective norm, and intention. Social cognitive theory, based on Bandura's cognitive learning approach to human action, emphasizes that individuals cannot successfully engage in safer sex if they perceive that they lack the ability to negotiate condom discussions. Interpersonal communication concepts call attention to the role that scripts, plans, and compliance-gaining play in dynamic communications about AIDS prevention. Functional theory helps explain why so many individuals—gay men and poor ethnic women (see chapter 4)—engage in unprotected sex that they know is risky.

Although the approaches described in this chapter have generated less research than cognitive decision models, they nonetheless offer insights into the rich, emotional nature of AIDS prevention choices and communication. In this way they extend knowledge about the social psychology of HIV infection.

CHAPTER FOUR

Culture, Poverty, and AIDS

Darlene Johson was born in Central Harlem in 1955, one of three children born to a mother who was chronically homeless, leaving her husband and children for long periods of time. . . . With no other means of support, Darlene lived with her abusive brother until after eleventh grade, when she married a "hardworking man." The couple soon had two children. . . . Things were often hard. The couple had many problems. Chief among them was their mutual passion, not for each other, but for heroin: "I didn't love him," she recalls. "He beat me, sometimes in front of the kids. It was drugs." After six years of abuse, Darlene found a way to leave . . . (and) met her second husband. This marriage was for love. Her husband, also a heroin user, worked. They had two sons. Her two older children also loved this man, and things were looking up.

Then her husband began to have high fevers and night sweats. He refused to go to the doctor, but Darlene knew it must be AIDS. By this time, she was tortured by the memory of all the times that she, her husband, and her stepbrother had shared needles. Darlene was tested and learned she was indeed HIV-positive.

Her husband died two months later. Alone with four children, Darlene was heartbroken: she had lost her husband, her stepbrother, and her stepfather in a single year. (Farmer, 1996, pp. 7–8)

Darlene's story is tragic, but all too common in inner-city neighborhoods. It is a compelling testament to the power that socioeconomic forces—poverty, drugs, racism, and sexism—exert on young men and women's AIDS-prevention behaviors. In this chapter, I examine the ways that society and culture influence safer sex behavior.

The present chapter departs from chapters 2 and 3 in its emphasis on broader macrosocial forces. Previous discussion focused on micropsychological and interpersonal communication factors like beliefs, affect, and compliance-gaining in dyads. Exploration of these factors is enormously useful. Yet the great strength of psychological and communication approaches—an emphasis on the individual or two-person unit—is also their greatest weakness. Individualistic approaches downplay the role that culture plays in influencing people's safer sex choices and constructions of social reality. Hortensia Amaro (1995), herself a psychologist, notes that traditional social psychological theories "ignore the way in which distal cultural forces and expectations as well as more immediate social norms and patterns in the individual's network and specific situational factors affect sexuality and sexual behaviors" (p. 440).

The key concept here is *culture,* defined by Cecil Helman (1990) as: **"a set of guidelines (both explicit and implicit) which individuals inherit as members of a particular society, and which tells them how to** *view* **the world, how to ex-perience it** *emotionally,* **and how to** *behave* **in it in relation to other people"** (pp. 2–3). If you reread this definition, you will see that this view of culture does not dismiss social psychology or interpersonal communication. On the contrary, it suggests that culture influences people's interpretations and experiences of life. Culture provides the structure for seeing the world. Psychological and commu-nication processes mediate culture. They provide the tools for representing and expressing cultural mores.

This chapter examines the effects of a variety of cultural influences on AIDS prevention behavior, beginning in the first section with the role that norms play in African American communities. In the second section, I examine the subtle ways that Latino culture influences gay men's sexual choices. The third portion focuses on the role that gender inequality plays in women's AIDS prevention decisions. The final section takes an internationalist perspective by briefly de-scribing the impact of cultural mores on sexual behavior in Africa.

AIDS IN AFRICAN AMERICAN COMMUNITIES

Although the death rate from AIDS is dropping in the U.S. population as a whole, the disease continues to devastate African American communities. African Ameri-cans constitute 12% of the U.S. population, but account for 37% of AIDS cases and an alarming 57% of all new reported cases of HIV infection (CDC, 1999a; Stolberg, 1998b). The disease is fast becoming an epidemic among low-income Blacks, whose higher rate of injection drug use and impoverished living condi-tions put them at risk to contract HIV. As Robert Fullilove (1995) observes:

> Urban poverty in the United States has created the perfect machinery for the con-tinued propagation of HIV. Inner-city poor neighborhoods often shelter a vigorous drug trade, numerous opportunities for strangers to engage in drug-mediated, unprotected sex, and numerous locations where these and other risk behaviors go virtually unchallenged. (p. 96)

There are many root and individual-level causes of these problems, but there is little doubt that a core explanation is societal prejudice.

Health Care and Culture

An important reason for the racial disparity in AIDS deaths is that the health care system still favors mainstream Whites over Blacks. This makes it difficult for Black people in the early stages of HIV infection to gain access to treatment or life-saving drugs. "It becomes an issue of trying to get someone to a specialist," said Dr. Robert G. Brooks, secretary of the Florida Health department. The problem, Brooks noted, is that a doctor who can treat poor Black patients is frequently miles away (Davis, 2000). Another problem is that the government was slow to respond as HIV infections dropped among gay men and began to spread rapidly through African American communities. Federal and state governments did not provide enough funds to educational and treatment centers serving poor Black residents.

At the same time, African American cultural norms encourage sexual adventurism that can put people at risk for HIV. African Americans engage in more polygamous sexual behaviors than Whites; they have sexual intercourse at an earlier age, more extramarital sex, and more sexual partners (Rushing, 1995). Some experts believe that these behaviors have their roots in the polygamous cultural traditions of West Africa, the ancestral home of many African Americans (Ruggles, 1994; Rushing, 1995, p. 118). In any event, Rushing (1995) notes, "the pattern is probably reinforced by sex-positive norms rooted in the poverty, drug subculture, and welfare dependence of the underclass, a disproportionate number of which consists of African Americans" (p. 118).

Men growing up in poor Black communities define manhood in macho terms (Oliver, 1989). A tough-guy refusal to use condoms may be attractive to young Black men inasmuch as it offers up a swaggering masculine self-concept that poverty and racism frequently foreclose. However, in the long run such a view of self is dysfunctional, and the preference for unsafe sex that it endorses greatly increases the likelihood of HIV infection for both these men and their female sexual partners.

Knowledge Deficits

Black Americans as a group are knowledgeable about AIDS transmission (Johnson, 1993; Sobo, 1995). Yet in low-income Black communities, people still harbor misconceptions. "There is still a disbelief that African Americans are at risk," says one inner-city AIDS education counselor. "A lot of people don't know how the virus is transmitted" (Stolberg, 1998b, p. 1). For example, African American adults with low education are somewhat less likely than their White counterparts to view condoms as effective methods to prevent HIV and are less cognizant of the HIV antibody test (Mays & Cochran, 1995; see also Hobfoll et al., 1993). There is more to these beliefs than simple cognitive deficits. Some low-income African Americans do not believe that condoms are effective because they harbor a generalized distrust of medical techniques recommended by the White establishment (Sobo, 1995). In order to understand the origins of this belief, we need to discuss the African American community context in more detail.

Community-Level Problems

One of the most serious barriers to AIDS prevention among African Americans is the widespread perception, which is changing as the rate of Black HIV infection increases, that AIDS does not affect African Americans but has its greatest impact on gay Whites. "Although individual African Americans were affected by HIV in the early 1980s," Paula Michal-Johnson and Sheryl Perlmutter Bowen (1992) note, "the larger African-American community denied existence of the disease and delayed prevention efforts" (p. 151). There are many reasons for this, including: (a) a perception that African Americans would be blamed for the disease and forced to cope with it on their own, (b) deep distrust of pronouncements from White government institutions, and (c) resentment that American society was telling Blacks what to do (Cochran & Mays, 1993; Dalton, 1989; Mitchell et al., 1997; Wingood & DiClemente, 1997). To some African Americans, campaigns to use condoms smacked of racism—an attempt of the larger society to reduce reproduction among Blacks (Weeks et al., 1995). Other African American leaders opposed needle-exchange programs, in which IDUs are provided with sterile needles and syringes without traces of HIV. Although there is no evidence that needle-exchange services increase drug use, some Black leaders opposed them, claiming they were in fact designed to keep Black addicts hooked on drugs (Donovan, 1999). At the same, time, broad conspiracy theories gained adherents in the Black community during the early 1990s. A significant minority of African Americans believed that AIDS was a genocidal racial plot (Rushing, 1995).

Although the genocidal notion seems ludicrous to many people and there is not one shred of scientific evidence to support a conspiracy theory (Sobo, 1995), it is easy to see how it could appeal to African American citizens with a historical memory for lynching and the notorious Tuskegee Experiment in which Blacks diagnosed with syphilis were never treated for the disease. In fact, as Rushing notes, "the records of other epidemics reveal that it is not uncommon for groups with high death rates from a mysterious disease to adopt irrational and paranoid views and to charge the government and other groups with conspiring to kill them off" (p. 158). During the cholera epidemic of the 1830s, poor Europeans believed they were the target of a frightful purge and accused government, the upper classes, and doctors of trying to poison them (Delaporte, 1986; Rushing, 1995). AIDS-risk denial may be a useful esteem-preserving strategy for the Black community. In the long run, however, it is not adaptive, particularly as infections among African Americans continue to rise.

Making matters more difficult, respected religious opinion leaders have traditionally taught that homosexuality is a sin and an abomination toward God (Fullilove & Fullilove, 1999). As a result of exposure to religious and other leaders' teachings, many inner-city Blacks have developed very hostile attitudes toward gays. As one Black man active in the Pentecostal Church said, "Why is it every time we came to church we gotta hear about faggots faggots lesbians dikes whores sissy bulldaggers—why couldn't we hear about the love of Christ?" (Fullilove & Fullilove, 1999, p. 1124). These views cause great discomfort to gay African Americans, making it difficult for them to feel positively about themselves, confide in family members, and seek social support. Such views have also contributed to the failure to stem the spread of AIDS within the Black community.

LATINO CULTURE AND HOMOSEXUALITY

Other cultural issues come to the fore in Hispanic communities, which also have been disproportionately affected by AIDS. Latinos account for 8% of the U.S. population but constitute an alarming 20% of new AIDS cases (CDC, 1999b). Latina women are at increasing risk to contract AIDS because of psychological and cultural factors that I discuss in detail in the next section. A particularly serious problem in this community is the high incidence of unprotected anal intercourse among Latino gay men. What's more, noted Rafael Díaz (1998) in his study of Latino gay men and HIV, "risk behavior continues to occur in the presence of substantial knowledge about HIV and AIDS, accurate perceptions of personal risk, and relatively strong intentions to practice safer sex" (p. 47). Many Latino gay men plan to engage in safer sex, but do not translate intentions into action. Díaz identifies four reasons why these patterns persist:

1. Widespread belief that Latino men have little control over sexual impulses. Latino culture drums into men the notion that sexual urges are powerful and based on strong biological needs that cannot or should not be contained. Men come to believe that "sexual arousal and rational decision-making processes cannot happen simultaneously within the person" (Díaz, 1998, p. 86). The machismo orientation of the culture is embodied in the sexual script that when sex gets hot, you keep going because that is the way sex is and this is the way men are constructed. Having internalized these cultural guidelines, many gay men find it difficult to carry out safer sex intentions, let alone formulate a condom use strategy.

2. Latino culture's emphasis on sexual penetration. Latino culture prizes success in sports, as well as fighting and boasting about sexual exploits, notably sexual penetration in heterosexual vaginal intercourse or gay anal sex. In a culture that emphasizes penetration by a "strong erect penis" and in which sexual activity without penetration is described as "nothing really happened," it is difficult to see how safer sex could measure up to the masculine ideal.

3. Family taboos regarding homosexuality. The culture places a strong emphasis on family relations—on individuals' loyalty and attachment to their nuclear and extended families. However, homosexuality is a taboo in many

families as parents consciously or unconsciously communicate the message that "homosexuals are failed men" (Díaz, 1998, p. 64; see also Singer et al., 1995). Desperate not to break relations with their family of origin, some Latino gay men keep silent about their homosexuality, even to the point of marrying women and engaging in same-sex affairs on the side. Afraid to disclose their gay identity to their parents, sexuality separated from the rest of their emotions, these men romanticize risky sex, somehow hoping it will fill the emotional void in their lives.

4. Sense of powerlessness. Experiences of poverty, racial prejudice, and a learned fatalism toward life leave many Latino gay men with a perception that they are powerless to change their lives. "How can we expect individuals who have little control over most of their lives' events to act with a great deal of agency and self-efficacy in the practice of safer sex?" Díaz asks (p. 121).

In psychological terms, at least some Latino gay men have low perceived behavioral control, little governing self-efficacy, weak subjective norms regarding safer sex, and little perceived ability to overcome prevailing sexual scripts. This has made it difficult for these men to practice safer sex, which in turn has led some to become infected with HIV.

WOMEN AND AIDS

Up to this point, the discussion has focused primarily on sociocultural origins of HIV infection among men. It is time to switch gears and discuss why women are increasingly at risk for diagnosis with the AIDS virus. AIDS cases have risen sharply among women, so much so that women throughout the world are being infected three times as quickly as men (Sobo, 1995). Women are primarily exposed to HIV through injection drug use and sexual intercourse with an HIV-infected male partner, who is frequently a drug addict himself (Amaro, 1995; Singer et al., 1995). The majority of female AIDS cases in the United States are young, poor women of color (Morokoff, Mays, & Coons, 1997; Wingood & DiClemente, 1998). Consider the story of Mildred, a 29-year-old daughter of a minister and mother of three, who recalls the day she discovered her husband was a heroin addict:

> I was in the bathroom, and I remember I was sitting on the toilet and there was one of those heaters on the wall. I don't know why, but I said, "I'm going to open that." I pulled it out and I found the needle, a cooker and the thing they tie themselves with, the rubber hose. When I saw that my heart went to my feet." (Connors, 1996, p. 91)

Mildred became infected with HIV, concluding that she "was going to die for having loved a heroin addict." It took her nearly 4 years to disclose her HIV infection. She used "one excuse after another to explain days spent depressed, sick in bed, and struggling to get to her job," notes Margaret Connors (1996, pp. 91–92). Mildred contracted meningitis, had 40 seizures, and weighed as little as 62 pounds at one point during her sickness. But thanks to the benefits of experimental drugs, she survived, her life becoming a "curious kind of waiting" (p. 92).

Mildred's story resembles those of thousands of other poor ethnic women. Study after study indicates that inner-city minority women ignore the risks and actively pursue behaviors that increase their chances of contracting HIV/AIDS. For example:

- More than 45% of sexually active low-income Black women from a San Francisco community reported that condoms were never used on any sexual occasion over the past 3 months (Wingood & DiClemente, 1998).
- Approximately half of a Providence, Rhode Island, sample of Latina adolescent mothers indicated that they rarely or never use a condom (Brown et al., 1998).
- More than 80% of a sample of impoverished minority female injection drug users or sex partners of drug users in Los Angeles had unprotected sex, and more than half of the female drug users shared their needles with other addicts (Nyamathi et al., 1995).
- In a qualitative study of primarily minority HIV-infected women from New York City, investigators found that many women confessed that they had delayed getting tested for months, even years (Siegel, Raveis, & Gorey, 1998).

How can we explain these findings? The discussion that follows attempts to answer this question, beginning with individual-level factors and moving to an examination of the impact of sociocultural forces, including how psychology, communication, and culture interact to influence unsafe sexual activities.

Lack of Knowledge

One reason why poor women of color fail to take precautions against HIV infection is they lack knowledge of AIDS. For example, some low-income women do not know that HIV-infected individuals can show no visible symptoms of illness, and assume that people infected with HIV know they have HIV (Sikkema et al., 1995). An HIV-positive Puerto Rican woman confessed she knew she could be at risk because she had never used a condom and had sexual intercourse with ex-addicts. However, she "never had a reason to suspect" she was infected because she was so healthy. "I mean, you know, I was working out 60 hours a month," she said. "I was going to school, I was working. I was the most active person . . . But I felt that my body was strong enough to deal with it" (Siegel et al., 1998, p. 119).

Poor ethnic women express other misconceptions. About one third of a sample of young adolescent mothers claimed that "the only people who are at risk are homosexuals, IV drug users, and people who received blood transfusions" (Brown et al., 1998, p. 569). This omits sexual partners of injecting drug users—a group to which many of these women may belong.

Low Perceived Susceptibility

The Health Belief Model suggests that perceived susceptibility to disease will motivate precautionary behavior. But as discussed in chapter 2, perceiving you are vulnerable to disease is a complex process. Although inner-city minority women have factual knowledge regarding the risks of unprotected sex and drug use, they frequently fail to connect this knowledge to their personal situations. Some women know drug abusers who have AIDS, but psychologically distance themselves from these individuals. Simple knowledge of the facts is not sufficient to overcome an illusion of invulnerability.

Poor women of color often do not perceive themselves to be at risk for HIV, although their behaviors put them objectively at risk to contract the virus (Hobfoll et al., 1993; Mays & Cochran, 1988; Sobo, 1995; St. Lawrence et al., 1998). Like other young people, inner-city women mistakenly believe they are not at risk because they are involved in a committed, monogamous relationship (Overby & Kegeles, 1994; St. Lawrence et al., 1998). In fact, their relationships frequently fit the pattern of serial monogamy.

Psychology of Poverty

Poverty, characterized as it is by the crippling effects of economic destitution, crime, drugs, and family chaos, powerfully influences HIV-related attitudes and coping strategies. In a discussion of minority women and AIDS, Vickie Mays and Susan Cochran (1988) offer a compassionate view of how poverty can alter perceptions of risk:

> Most women, particularly when their life reality is that of being poor, Black, Latina, or outside the law through drug abuse or street prostitution, have always lived with risks of some kind. AIDS is simply one more risk with which to be concerned. These women have long histories of facing omnipresent dangers not often experienced by the middle class and mustering what scarce resources exist to cope with these dangers. . . . The key to poor ethnic women's response to AIDS is their perception of its danger relative to the hierarchy of other risks present in their lives and the existence of resources available to act differently. Competition for these women's attention includes more immediate survival needs, such as obtaining shelter for the night, securing personal safety or safety of their children, or interfacing with the governmental system in order to obtain financial resources. For women who often, realistically, feel powerless to change the external realities of their lives—where they live, how much they earn, or the system's rules for getting financial supplements—AIDS may be of relatively low concern. (p. 951)

Earlier I argued that individuals (e.g., low-income ethnic women) deny susceptibility to AIDS because it is psychologically functional to do so. The larger perspective of Mays and Cochran suggests another explanation: AIDS is only one of many terrible risks to which minority women are exposed. In order to assign AIDS high personal priority, they must mentally allocate it a place on their psychological agendas. Unfortunately, their emotional plates are so full that they are unable to accomplish this important task.

A related view is offered by Connors (1992). Her research focuses on drug users' risk-taking behavior and is highly relevant to perceptions of risk among inner-city women, many of whom abuse drugs. Connors notes that after a time "routine risk taking becomes habitual." Eventually the level of risk involved in activities ranging from purchasing drugs to engaging in unprotected sex becomes rationalized—"downgraded through routine" (p. 596). Having lost the capacity to shock the individual, these activities become habitual, part of a cycle of increasing risk, distorted perceptions, and more risk, until finally the unthinkable—AIDS—afflicts the individual and she wakes up, too late, hoping to recapture her life.

Drug Addiction

Drug addiction takes a large toll on low-income women of color. More than half of the African American and Latina IDUs surveyed by Adeline Nyamathi and her colleagues (1995) reported that they shared needles and syringes, behaviors that greatly increase the risk of HIV infection. More than 60% of these women indicated that they did not clean needles (to remove HIV) because they did not have their own needle, and 57% said they did not disinfect needles because alcohol or bleach was not available. Planned behavior theory suggests that when people lack the resources to implement behaviors, intention will not predict action. In this case, poverty and federal government opposition to needle-exchange programs also make it difficult for women (and men, for that matter) who intend to clean needles to actually do so.

While male drug users engage in risky behaviors, Connors (1992) argues that female injection drug users take more HIV risks than men. Noting that women have less money to buy drugs and are less likely to pull robberies to get cash, she says that women use prostitution to gain money, which increases their risk for HIV infection (see also Logan, Leukefeld, & Farabee, 1998). Moreover, because women place a higher premium on connecting socially with other people than do men (Amaro, 1995), they are more inclined to lend someone a needle or borrow a needle to get high with a fellow user.

Gender Inequality and Socialization

According to gender-specific approaches to AIDS prevention, women's inequality with respect to income, social status, and interpersonal power places them at

a serious disadvantage in communicating about safer sex and taking other precautions against HIV infection (Amaro, 1995; Cline & McKenzie, 1996; Wingood & DiClemente, 1997, 1998). Theorists also argue that as a result of sex-
role socialization, low-income women are unduly concerned with serving others and insufficiently attentive to their own personal needs.

Economic Forces.   Inequities in wages and job opportunities can leave women
dependent on men for economic resources. "As the economic disparity between
men and women increases and favors men," Gina Wingood and Ralph DiClemente (1998) point out, "women may be more susceptible to direct or indirect
financial incentives to actually engage in high-risk sex" (p. 32). Wingood and
DiClemente found that women who received most of their income from Aid
to Families with Dependent Children (AFDC) were significantly more likely to
report not using condoms over the past 3 months than women who were employed. Dependent on men for money to supplement AFDC payments, these
minority women may have felt they had no choice but to comply with men
when they wanted unprotected sex.

Economic factors influence women's relationship choices, which can place
them at increased risk for contracting AIDS. Many poor ethnic women stand a
good chance of forming relationships with men who use injection drugs, in view
of the heavy drug use in minority communities (Worth, 1989). In other cases,
money gets tied to risky sex through heroin use. Connors (1996) notes that:

> Drug users typically have "running partners"—people who shoot up together,
> scam, and generally spend time together. Drug-using women prefer male running
> partners for the protection they afford. But men prefer not to run with women
> and would rather have sexual relationships with "good" (non-drug using) women.
> Therefore, women tend to go to great lengths to secure a male running partner,
> which often entails increased needle sharing, sex for protection, and for access to
> drugs. (p. 96)

Although economic factors affect women's unsafe sex choices, they are not
the only—nor necessarily most important—influence. As Elisa Sobo (1995)
notes in an elegant analysis of poor women and AIDS, "most women do not
perceive their own participation in condomless sex as purchased by men, nor do
they generally see it as forced upon them by a need for men's money" (p. 75). To
understand why women choose unsafe sex, as Sobo put it, we need to look at
other sociocultural factors.

Sexual Power.   Feminist theorists argue that women's unequal social status,
along with socialization to adopt a passive and subservient gender role, discourages low-income women from taking the initiative in the arena of safer sex
(Amaro, 1995; Wingood & DiClemente, 1998). There is evidence that poor
Black women do not perceive that they have the power to make a male partner

use a condom, particularly when the man resists their request (Wingood &
DiClemente, 1998; Wingood, Hunter-Gamble, & DiClemente, 1993).

Women's limited power in negotiating condom use is particularly evident in
physically abusive relationships. African American women who are involved
with physically abusive partners are less likely to use condoms than women
whose partners are not abusive (Stevens & Bogart, 1999; Wingood & DiClemente, 1998). One woman interviewed by Wingood and her colleagues (1993)
disclosed that her partner responded in this manner when she mentioned condom use: "B___, I'll beat your a___! Don't do me like that" [don't ask me to
wear a condom].

Another woman confided that "I never have [asked my partner to use a con-
dom], I'm scared to tell him to use one, he ain't been using no condom . . . you
don't know my man, honey" (p. 199). For these reasons, many women find it
easier to talk with partners about their drug injection practices than about condom use (Wermuth, Ham, & Robbins, 1992).

Culture interacts with sexual power in dynamic ways. Latina women are
taught to play a submissive role in sexual relationships, bear children, and respect the male partner, who traditionally believes that only unprotected sex
constitutes "real sex" (Díaz, 1998; Marin et al., 1998; Weeks et al., 1995). A con-
tradictory strain in Latina culture is an emphasis on women's psychological
strength, strong drive, and determination (Singer et al., 1995). As a result, increasing numbers of Hispanic women are asserting themselves against abusive
sex partners. Yet "the duality of gender socialization" causes some to throw
drug-addicted, sexually unfaithful husbands out of the house while still engaging in risky sexual activities with them (Singer et al., p. 99).

Gender-Role Socialization.   Gender approaches argue that women's self-esteem is grounded in interpersonal relationships—in forging strong connections
between self and others (Amaro, 1995; Miller, 1986). The problem, feminist theorists maintain, is that "women are taught that their main goal in life is to serve
others—first men, and later, children" (Miller, p. 62). This makes women unduly
reluctant to challenge men to practice safer sex, as they fear that these behaviors
would disrupt a valued romantic relationship.

Arguing that sexism and poverty make it difficult for women to construct a
healthy self-concept on their own, Sobo argues that women "require a heterosexual relationship with a man" to gain social status and emotional fulfillment
(1995, p. 102). Women, she notes, have been taught that sex should be part of a
loving relationship, in which both partners trust one another completely. Condom use undermines this trust and tugs at the fabric of the idealized monogamous relationship, what Sobo calls "the monogamy narrative." As researcher
Dooley Worth (1989) observes:

> Condoms for many individuals are symbols of extra-relationship activity. The
> subconscious message their presentation for use delivers is: "You are not the only

one with whom I am having sex." Individuals generally do not want to be re-minded of this, as it raises too many painful questions and issues that are often not discussed. (p. 304)

And so, the theory suggests, in order to maintain (what is frequently) a fan-tasy—"I love my man and he loves me back"—women perform mental and behavioral gymnastics. They deny that men are cheating, minimize their sus-ceptibility to HIV, and practice unsafe sex. To acknowledge the truth would be to admit that the life and self-concept they have built around a man is a fiction and that the status they have achieved in their social circle is a sham. So they reject condoms, not because they are ignorant of AIDS but because they don't want to burst their bubble or do anything that would threaten a relationship that sustains them psychologically.

In some cases, women's need to believe in a trusting relationship prevents them from recognizing tell-tale signs of deception. One woman said that after she tested positive, her boyfriend revealed he had known he was infected with HIV. He defended his decision not to tell her, claiming "I figured when you learned to love me we could die together" (Siegel et al., 1998, p. 120).

Other minority women resist using condoms because of their cultural con-notations. These women view condoms not just as contraceptive devices, but as social stigmas—negative symbols of women's sexuality (Worth, 1989; see also Wilson et al., 1993). Proposing condom use means a woman is sexually available and "out for sex." In many communities, Worth points out, "such associations violate traditional normative behavior, which dictates that women play a pas-sive sexual role. A woman who suggests using a condom can be perceived as deviating from the cultural norm, resulting in the loss of her sexual desirability and social status" (p. 303).

Perhaps this sounds sexist, reaffirming a traditional view of women as emo-tional, passive, and dependent on men. Feminist theorists would respond that society and inner-city culture have left women with few other ways to build their self-esteem (e.g., Amaro, 1995; Sobo, 1995). African American women may be particularly tempted to "put their lives in men's hands" in light of the shortage of young Black men in inner-city communities, lost through AIDS, death, and imprisonment (Worth, 1989, p. 302).

For these reasons, poor ethnic women choose unsafe sex, no doubt project-ing onto it their hopes and misconceptions simultaneously. As Sobo notes, im-plicitly adopting a functional theory approach, "unsafe sex provides women— particularly those dependent on relations with men for status and self-esteem— with a way to feel good about their lives" (p. 107).

Individual Differences

So far I have played up the implications of gender and culture, de-emphasizing the effects of psychological factors on women's AIDS prevention decisions.

However, culture gains its power from the way that people experience social structural constraints and internalize global values. Macrosocial factors like poverty, racism, and sexism are significant psychologically because they influence values, attitudes, and identifications.

As powerful as culture is, its imprint differs, depending on the background and personality of the individual. Women who feel hopeless and have low self-esteem or self-efficacy are not apt to insist on safer sex or discuss condoms with partners (Jemmott et al., 1995; Sobo, 1995). Those who have been beaten down by drugs, sexual abuse, or poverty and have become "psychologically vanquished"—that is, have lost the ability to cope effectively with stress—seem to be particularly likely to engage in risky sexual behaviors.

Not everyone fits this bill. Not all women succumb. Women are less likely to engage in risky sexual and drug-injection behaviors when they have a stronger self-concept, better coping skills, higher self-efficacy, and greater social support (Jemmott & Jemmott, 1992; Jemmott et al., 1995). For reasons we do not totally understand, some women from impoverished backgrounds develop the psychological wherewithal to protect themselves from HIV infection, whereas others find it difficult to extricate themselves emotionally from the vicious cycle of drug addiction, sexual exploitation, and subservience.

Summary

Although gender perspectives have significantly advanced knowledge of AIDS prevention behavior, like all approaches they have shortcomings. Research generated by gender-based perspectives tends to focus exclusively on women, making it difficult to know whether some problems experienced by low-income females (e.g., low self-efficacy, poor communication skills) are worse than those of low-income males. In addition, gender power approaches do not tell us why certain women take precautions against AIDS and others don't, or why some women insist that men enact safer sex strategies whereas others are more submissive. Yet these are rectifiable problems, ones that no doubt will be dealt with as more research on gender issues is conducted.

Gender-specific perspectives provide a useful antidote to the field's preoccupation with men's unsafe sex behavior. Given the dramatic upsurge in HIV infection among women and the fact that AIDS afflicts a panoply of women—running the gamut from inner-city Blacks to rural Whites (Belluck, 1998) to residents of many African countries—an analysis of the role that gender plays in the psychology of AIDS prevention seems long overdue.

RISKY SEX ABROAD: THE CASE OF AFRICA

Durban, South Africa—Mercy Makhalemele found out she was HIV-positive when she was pregnant with her second child. She was 23, had been married for five years, and was faithful to her husband. She cried all the way home from the prenatal clinic, but was too afraid to tell anyone for nearly a year.

When she finally did tell her husband, he beat her to the ground, knocking her against a lighted stove and badly burning her wrist, she said. Then he threw her out of the house, refusing to believe that he had given her the virus. The next day, he went to the shoe store she managed. With everyone watching, he shouted at her to collect all her things, he would have nothing to do with someone with HIV, the virus that causes AIDS.

Her employers dismissed her that afternoon . . .

It is hard to find anyone who publicly admits to being HIV-positive. Many go to their graves with their secret, so great is the stigma. . . . The shame that people feel and the treatment they suffer at the hands of their communities has far-reaching consequences for efforts to fight the spread of the virus and treat the sick, experts say. For one thing, it keeps people from wanting to find out whether they have AIDS, and it encourages even those who know they are infected to act as everyone else does, and perhaps even spread the disease. (Daley, 1998, p. 1)

Such is the tragedy of AIDS in eastern and southern Africa, where as many as one in every four people is infected with HIV (Daley, 1998). In Uganda, where rich and poor are equally affected, one tenth of the population—1.7 million people—have reportedly contracted the virus (Nyakabwa, 1997; see also Box 4.1). Unlike the United States, the infection is spread primarily through heterosexual intercourse—an act that is prized and encouraged through prostitution, rampant adultery, and wife-sharing.

Africa is not the only continent where HIV infection is devastating cities and crippling economies. More than one third of new HIV infections occurred in Southeast Asian countries, such as Cambodia and Thailand, and the infection rate is growing (Morisky & Coan, 1998; Steinfatt & Mielke, 1999; see Table 4.1). However, Africa has been particularly hard hit, and the psychological dimensions of AIDS in Africa have been well documented. Thus, the following discussion focuses on the African context, offering an overview—a thumbnail sketch—of the vast literature on this subject, drawing on Rushing's (1995) work on this topic. Chapter 6 offers a discussion of AIDS prevention campaigns in Thailand.

Sex and Culture

In most African societies, sex is viewed positively, as an essential form of recreation between lovers, casual acquaintances, and even adulterers. Polygamy is widespread and sanctioned (Rushing, 1995). What's more, wives gain respect in kinship units or clans based on the number of children they bear. This reduces the strength of emotional bonds between husbands and wives, which in turn makes it easier for spouses (particularly men) to engage in extramarital sex.

Men have abundant freedom to engage in premarital and extramarital sexual relationships. In a variety of countries, men routinely visit their extramarital

---

BOX 4.1

AIDS IN AFRICA: A TRAGEDY OF INCOMPARABLE PROPORTIONS

In Africa, AIDS is a time bomb waiting to go off. Thousands have died already, and with HIV infection rates climbing, the disease is expected to wipe out hundreds of thousands, even millions, more. In South Africa alone, AIDS is expected to kill six times as many people as were killed by atomic bombs in Hiroshima and Nagasaki (Sternberg, 1999a). These statistics, accumulated by UNAIDS, the World Health Organization, and the U.S. Department of State and reported alongside Sternberg's article, tell the disquieting story.

South Africa
   Population: 49.2 million
   HIV infection rate: Ranges from 7% to 37%
   People living with HIV: 2.9 million
   Projected AIDS deaths, 2010: 4.4 million

Zambia
   Population: 9 million
   HIV infection rate: Roughly 20%
   People living with HIV: 770,000
   Projected AIDS deaths, 2010: 4.2 million

Zimbabwe
   Population: 12 million
   HIV infection rates: 35% urban, 20% rural
   People living with HIV: 1.5 million
   Projected AIDS deaths, 2010: 4.5 million

Uganda
   Population: 19 million
   HIV infection rate: 15%
   People living with HIV: 930,000
   Projected AIDS deaths, 2010: 6.3 million

From Sternberg (1999a).

---

partners on the way home from work, making a daily stop at what some men jokingly call their "second office" (Ungar, 1989, p. 475). As Rushing observes:

> In contrast to Americans, who usually view sex morally and think that people who have multiple partners (even if unmarried) are immoral and unfaithful, most Africans do not judge sexual behavior in such terms at all. They experience little guilt about sex, and they enter into sex more casually and have more sexual partners than Westerners do. (1995, p. 62)

Many of the same power inequities that operate in poor American communities are at work in African societies. In many cultures, a woman must obey her

TABLE 4.1
HIV Infection, Region by Region

Region	Total with HIV/AIDS	Infected in 1998	Percentage of Adults Infected	Modes of Transmission
Sub-Saharan Africa	22.5 million	4.0 million	8.00	HS
North Africa, Middle East	210,000	19,000	.13	IDU, HS
South & Southeast Asia	6.7 million	1.2 million	.69	HS
East Asia & Pacific	560,000	200,000	.068	IDU, HS, MSM
Latin America	1.4 million	160,000	.57	MSM, IDU, HS
Caribbean	330,000	45,000	1.96	HS, MSM
Eastern Europe & Central Asia	270,000	80,000	.14	IDU, MSM
Western Europe	500,000	30,000	.25	MSM, IDU
North America	890,000	44,000	.56	MSM, IDU, HS
Australia & New Zealand	12,000	600	.10	MSM, IDU

Note. HS = Heterosexual sex; IDU = Intravenous drug use; MSM = Men having sex with men. From UNAIDS. New York Times, November 24, 1998, p. D7.

husband, bear as many children as her husband wants, and take responsibility for raising the kids. Women who cannot have children face disgrace and ostracism.

Sex may be viewed as a positive form of recreation between casual acquaintances in many African societies, but it is still a man's world when it comes to sexual relationships (Obbo, 1995). In most African countries, it is socially acceptable for married men to have mistresses and concubines; some societies permit wife-sharing, where a wife has sex with individuals other than her husband, typically a distant relative of the husband's tribe (Rushing, 1995). Children who are born from these sexual dalliances become part of the husband's kinship group, which provides an additional incentive for men to have extramarital relations.

The desire to create offspring has a negative impact on condom use. As a young man from Kenya said bluntly, "Use of condoms is not appropriate because it is like throwing one's children away" (Cameron, Witte, & Nzyuko, 1999, p. 160).

Stereotyped beliefs about sexuality also act as impediments to safer sex. In Kenya, the sexual urge is believed to be "strong—at times uncontrollable" (Blair et al., 1997, p. 51). Some Kenyan men incorrectly believe that condoms are ineffective because they fail to take into account "the sexual superiority of the African man," whose "erection power" is thought to be so strong that it would cause American-manufactured condoms to burst (Cameron et al., 1999, p. 158). This belief, based on a primitive theory of African sexual culture, undoubtedly reduces men's enthusiasm for using condoms.

Noting their sex drive is strong, some Kenyan men say they can persevere with condoms during the early hours of the night, but "by midnight they insist on skin-to-skin" (Witte, Cameron, & Nzyuko, 1996, p. 19). In eastern Africa, prostitutes typically have sex with clients at least six times a night; unfortunately, condoms come only in packs of three (K. Witte, personal communication, August 17, 1999).

African women, for their part, can view sex as a way to escape physically grueling work or to gain independence from oppressive male control. Women may sell sex for money or become sexually involved with men other than their husbands, who they hope will provide money and opportunities for economic security (Rushing, 1995).

Many of these women engage in unprotected sex. Although impoverished American prostitutes frequently use condoms (Sobo, 1995), commercial sex workers in Kenya are reluctant to suggest condom use. "Here it is not easy for a woman to face a man and tell him to use a condom," one female sex worker told Kenzie Cameron and her associates (1999, p. 153). "We are women, we are weak and shy, we cannot ask them to use condoms," another sex worker said.

Summary

AIDS would probably not have emerged as a full-blown epidemic in Africa had there not been a mixing of people from different tribes and cultures. With urbanization came the greater possibility for individuals afflicted with HIV to spread the virus to others through polygamous sex. Rampant prostitution, sexual relationships between people of different tribes, and increased opportunities for women to escape male domination by engaging in extramarital sex also helped facilitate the spread of AIDS in Africa.

Had safer sex practices been followed, the rate of HIV infection would undoubtedly be lower. But, as discussed earlier, many African men and women find condoms incompatible with sexual and cultural norms. Moreover, those who would like to use condoms often find them unavailable (Cameron et al., 1999). HIV testing is also not available in many areas. Nor are new drugs that can increase the life span of those infected with HIV. And even where testing or drugs are accessible, women frequently shy away from taking advantage of such services, fearing they will be stigmatized or ostracized (Daley, 1998).

INTEGRATING CULTURE, COMMUNICATION, AND PSYCHOLOGY

This chapter has argued that we cannot understand or prevent HIV infection without considering culture, ethnicity, and gender. But behavior is complex. A comprehensive analysis of cultural influences on HIV prevention behavior requires that we examine both culture and the ways that microlevel social psychological and communication factors mediate sociocultural effects (see Fig. 4.1).

For example, culturally oriented research finds that in the United States, low-income people of color are knowledgeable about AIDS prevention but fail to

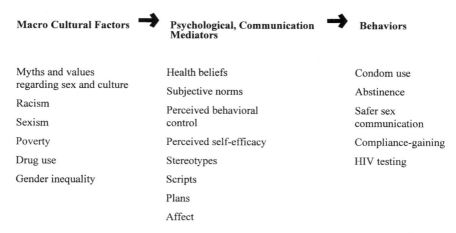

FIG. 4.1.   Model of culture, psychology, and AIDS prevention.

translate this knowledge into action. The theory of reasoned action helps explain why (e.g., Jemmott & Jemmott, 1991). The TRA emphasizes that knowledge is not likely to lead to changes in behavioral intentions unless it influences key beliefs and subjective norms. A person can know that unprotected sex is dangerous, but intend to do it anyway because she believes that it will offer pleasure, provide drug money, or prevent a traumatizing argument with a sexual partner. Another individual may engage in risky behaviors, despite knowing the risks, because he believes these activities are endorsed—or at least not condemned—by influential others in the community.

Other individual-oriented approaches also can be usefully combined with macro cultural perspectives. For example, the Health Belief Model calls attention to the fact that, for many poor minority women, unsafe sex offers more benefits—in terms of rewards to the self-concept and relationship security—than costs, despite the objective risks posed by unprotected sexual intercourse. In addition, the theory of planned behavior suggests that some individuals—for example, promiscuous Latino gay men, sexually active Kenyan heterosexuals, and poor, drug-abusing women—do not view sex as being under volitional control. Intention to practice safer sex will not accurately forecast behavior for these individuals. Their behavior may be better explained by sexual scripts or affect. Social cognitive theory suggests that poor ethnic women may not try to convince their male partners to use condoms because they feel they lack skill in initiating a conversation. Functional perspectives remind us that before we criticize low-income women for engaging in unsafe sex, we should understand the many psychosocial benefits such sex promises. Finally, interpersonal communication concepts suggest that one reason women here and abroad do not make concerted efforts to gain safer-sex compliance is that they invoke cultural scripts that prescribe sexual passivity.

CONCLUSION

By considering the role that culture and gender play in HIV prevention, we gain increased insight into AIDS prevention behavior.

Cultural approaches call attention to the role that knowledge deficits, social norms, racism, and community-level denial play in the etiology of AIDS in ethnic communities, particularly poor Black neighborhoods. Family taboos and cultural myths exert an important impact on Latino gay men's unsafe-sex decisions. A host of socioeconomic and gender power factors influence low-income minority women's AIDS precautionary behaviors. Poverty and drug abuse lead women to minimize the risks of HIV infection. Inequalities in job opportunities leave women dependent on men for economic resources, which can place them at the mercy of sexually irresponsible or physically abusive men. However, coercion (either direct or indirect) is not the only factor that causes poor women to have unsafe sex. Discouraged or effectively prevented by society from actualizing themselves through their own cognitive or social achievements, some women depend on men for emotional gratifications. Condom use can threaten a heterosexual relationship and counters the idealized monogamous narrative that sustains some minority women. Thus to preserve a relationship and their own self-esteem, minority women frequently choose unsafe sex (Sobo, 1995).

In southeastern Africa, sexual mores, gender stratification, and gender-role stereotypes operate powerfully to discourage men and women from practicing safer sex. This has led to epidemic-level HIV infection that, in 2000, shows no sign of stopping.

Culture does not simply stamp its effect on people. By understanding the subtle ways that culture weaves its "psychological spell" on people in poor areas of the United States and abroad, we can better devise ways to undo its sorcery, thereby helping people protect themselves against HIV infection.

CHAPTER FIVE

Applying Persuasion Theories to AIDS Prevention

An ancient Chinese proverb states that "a journey of a thousand miles begins with a single step." It could be the guiding description of persuasion. Contrary to popular opinion, persuasion does not happen with the flick of a switch. You cannot just get someone to change his or her mind. On the contrary, persuasion is a process that takes time, consists of a number of steps, and actively involves the recipient of the message. If a communicator wants to persuade people to change their minds about an issue, he or she must "get into the target audience's heads," understand how they think about issues, appreciate their mental hang-ups, empathize with their private fears, and gear the message accordingly.

This is particularly true in the area of AIDS prevention, which involves persuading people about sex, one of life's most pleasurable activities, but one freighted with emotion and risk. AIDS also brings to mind the possibility of death, stigmatized groups, loss of loved ones, and making behavioral changes that many people would rather not consider. AIDS educators cannot snap their fingers and get people to abstain from risky sex. Nothing in life—least of all persuading people to change sexual habits—is that easy.

And yet the fact that safer sex persuasion is difficult does not mean it is impossible. Quite the contrary. When faced with difficult challenges, the human mind shows uncommon flexibility and adaptive strength. This is abundantly clear in the area of AIDS prevention, where there have been numerous success stories—many instances of interventions and communication campaigns that have produced major shifts in attitudes and behavior toward unprotected sex (Kalichman, 1998). And although much work needs to be done, as was evident from the discussion in chapters 2 through 4, there is every reason to believe that systematic application of theory to AIDS prevention campaigns will help us design more effective programs to help people protect themselves against HIV infection.

This chapter examines the ways that persuasion theories can be used to influence AIDS precautionary attitudes and behaviors. Chapter 6 continues this discussion, focusing on communication campaigns.

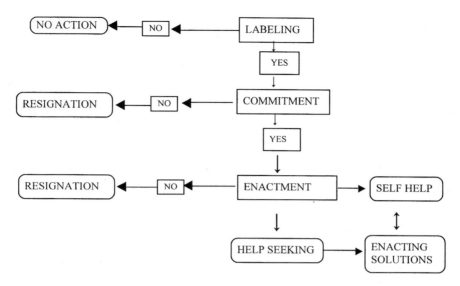

FIG. 5.1.   The AIDS Risk Reduction Model (ARRM).

STAGE MODELS

The AIDS Risk Reduction Model (ARRM) postulates a three-stage process whereby people modify AIDS preventive behaviors (Catania, Kegeles, & Coates, 1990; see Fig. 5.1). During the first—critical—stage, individuals must label their risky behaviors as problematic. The model correctly recognizes that before people can make enduring changes in attitudes or behaviors, they must recognize that their actions put them at risk for contracting HIV. The second stage is commitment. Once individuals label their behaviors as risky, they must make a commitment to reduce unsafe sexual behaviors and to engage in less risky actions. During the third stage, enactment, people begin taking steps to change behavior. Social support and constructive communication between partners can help individuals accomplish these goals.

A second approach, the transtheoretical model, assumes that people progress through five stages of change (Prochaska, DiClemente, & Norcross, 1992). In the first stage, **precontemplation**, individuals have no desire to change their behavior. As G. K. Chesterton said, "It isn't that they can't see the solution. It is that they can't see the problem" (Prochaska et al., 1992, p. 1103). The second step is **contemplation**, in which people recognize they have a problem and are considering making a change within the next 6 months. During the third phase, **preparation**, individuals are actively planning to change and have even taken steps toward reducing the problematic behaviors. The fourth stage, **action**, occurs when people actually modify risky behaviors, and **maintenance** is the stage in which people sustain behavioral changes over a long period of time.

The model recognizes—indeed assumes—that people relapse, regress to earlier stages, and recycle through stages several times before maintaining long-term change. It accepts as a given an observation made by Mark Twain a century ago: "Habit is habit, and not to be flung out of the window, but coaxed downstairs a step at a time" (cited in Prochaska et al., 1994, p. 471). According to the transtheoretical view, persuasive communications must be tailored to the needs of people at a particular stage. For example, messages directed at precontemplators try to convince them that their behaviors put them at risk, whereas communications geared to contemplators encourage them to. consider substituting a new behavior for the risky activity (Maibach & Cotton, 1995).

A third approach combines stages of change with persuasive communication theory. According to William McGuire (1985), persuasion can be viewed as a series of input and output steps. In Fig. 5.2, the input column labels refer to standard persuasion variables out of which a message can be constructed. The output row headings refer to the steps that individuals must be persuaded to take if the message is to have its intended impact.

As the figure shows, a message must clear many hurdles if it is to succeed in influencing attitudes and behavior. An AIDS prevention communication may not clear the first hurdle—exposure—because it never reaches the target audience or alternatively because receivers, finding the message threatening, tune it out as soon as they view it. Or a safer sex campaign message may pass the first few steps but get knocked out of the box when it threatens deeper values.

More optimistically, the input–output matrix views success as a multidimensional concept. Campaigns are frequently designed simply to get people to think about changing their attitudes (Step 3), to improve safer sex communication skills (Step 5), as well as to influence more long-term behaviors (Steps 10–12).

This model is a useful schema for discussing AIDS preventive communications. This chapter and the one that follows are organized around the model's major input factors: source, message, channels, and receivers. Output factors are called on in describing the nature of message effects.

SOURCE FACTORS

Ever since Aristotle, communicators have recognized that ethos or credibility of the source is a key factor in persuasion. "We believe good men more fully and more readily than others," Aristotle wrote (Roberts, 1954, pp. 24–25). But the Greek sage did not explicate what he meant by "good," leaving it to contemporary researchers to spell out specific aspects of the concept of source credibility.

Research indicates that credibility consists primarily of two components: expertise and trustworthiness (Perloff, 1993). Communicators who are perceived

INPUT: Independent (Communication) Variables / OUTPUT: Dependent Variables (Response Steps Mediating Persuasion)	SOURCE (number, unanimity, demographics, attractiveness, credibility ••)	MESSAGE (type appeal, type information, inclusion/omission, organization, repetitiveness ••)	CHANNEL (modality, directness, context ••)	RECEIVER (demographics, ability, personality, life style ••)	DESTINATION (immediacy/delay, prevention/cessation, direct/immunization •)
1. Exposure to the communication					
2. Attending to it					
3. Liking, becoming interested in it					
4. Comprehending it (learning what)					
5. Skill acquisition (learning how)					
6. Yielding to it (attitude change)					
7. Memory storage of content and /or agreement					
8. Information search and retrieval					
9. Deciding on basis of retrieval					
10. Behaving in accord with decision					
11. Reinforcement of desired acts					
12. Post-behavioral consolidating					

FIG. 5.2.   The communication/persuasion model as an input–output matrix. From "Theoretical foundations of campaigns" (p. 304), by W. J. McGuire. In R. E. Rice and C. K. Atkin (Eds.), *Public Communication Campaigns*, 1989, Thousand Oaks, CA: Sage.

to be experts and are seen as trustworthy can influence attitudes. The Surgeon General's (1988) brochure "Understanding AIDS" is an example of a message that attempted to change attitudes by making expertise salient to audience members. The U.S. Surgeon General is a recognized expert on medicine and health.

Expertise alone is not sufficient to change attitudes. People may distrust experts or discount the communicator's expertise. Thus, communicators should also rely on trustworthiness, showing that they mean what they say and say what they mean. One way that sources can promote trustworthiness is through similarity, or by convincing message recipients that they share their values, morals, or background characteristics.

Trustworthiness and similarity are likely to be especially important in communicating with low-income minority respondents, who frequently distrust mainstream authorities. Kalichman and Coley (1995) showed that an HIV education videotape exerted the strongest impact on poor African American women's intention to get tested for HIV when the message was delivered by an African American female. Unfortunately, few media messages directed at urban minorities focus on source–receiver similarity. "Usually when someone of authority on the screen talks about the risks of AIDS," Mays and Cochran (1988) note, "this individual is a White male, not an ethnic minority member, and seldom an ethnic woman" (p. 951).

Another factor that enhances trustworthiness is a perception that the speaker has converted from an opposing set of beliefs to the cause of AIDS prevention. Convert communicators are individuals who have converted from one lifestyle or ideology to a totally different set of beliefs (Perloff, 1993). Such individuals can be highly persuasive. Consider the case of Rebekka Armstrong, former *Playboy* Playmate, who liked to party and have unprotected sex when she was a teenager. Rebekka, now HIV-positive, believes she contracted HIV when she was 16, from sexual intercourse with a male model. After years of suffering, denial, and drug abuse, Armstrong has gone public with her infection, trying to teach young people the dangers of unprotected sex. She recently spoke to a capacity crowd at Cleveland State University, touching the hearts of many who attended the speech. She is a classic convert communicator, whose credibility is undoubtedly enhanced by her physical appeal. "If someone this beautiful can get HIV," people may reason, "it's obviously not just the ugly 'low-lifes' who get it." This may induce some young people to question their own perceived invulnerability to infection.

Celebrity Sources: The Case of Magic Johnson

"It's God's way," Magic Johnson said in 1991 when he announced he was HIV-positive. "He is now directing me to become a teacher to carry the message about AIDS to everyone. I think I can spread the message about AIDS better than almost anyone" (Penner & Fritzsche, 1993, p. 1035).

Earvin "Magic" Johnson is the quintessential celebrity spokesperson for HIV prevention. As an attractive, superstar professional basketball player, he was well known and well liked by millions when he announced on November 7, 1991 that he had tested positive for HIV. His announcement was front-page news and a lead item in news broadcasts across the land. The media lionized him at first, calling him a hero, praising his positive, optimistic outlook, and heralding him as a superstar spokesperson for AIDS awareness (Payne & Mercuri, 1993). "A hero exits with a smile," a *San Francisco Examiner* headline proclaimed. Although follow-up stories took a more critical stance, suggesting that Johnson may have contracted the virus through wildly promiscuous sex, the bulk of the coverage of Johnson during the weeks following his announcement was positive, reflecting the media and public's admiration for his courage in disclosing his condition and dedication to educate young people about AIDS. From a persuasion perspective, the question is: Did this celebrity source change HIV-related attitudes or behavior?

Johnson's announcement stimulated public interest in AIDS. More than 1.7 million calls streamed into the National AIDS Hotline during the 2 months following his announcement. Compare this number to 7,372—the number of calls placed during the 3-month period prior to his disclosure (Kalichman, 1994). African American men were most likely to call, suggesting that source–receiver similarity was at work (see Fig. 5.3; and also see Moskowitz, Binson, & Catania, 1997). Requests for HIV antibody testing also increased dramatically during the 20 days after the disclosure (Kalichman, 1998). However, these personal concerns did not lead to major readjustments in people's perceptions of vulnerability to HIV. There is limited evidence that perceptions of personal risk increased after Johnson's announcement. People may have defensively denied that they

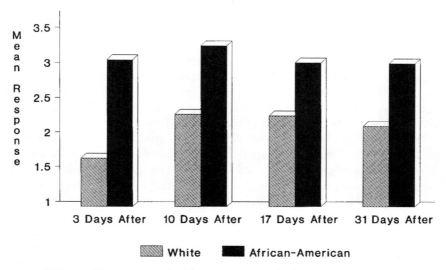

FIG. 5.3. Mean responses for African American and White men to an item addressing concern about AIDS following Magic Johnson's announcement at four post-announcement assessment points. From *Preventing AIDS: A Sourcebook for Behavioral Interventions* (p. 158), by S. C. Kalichman, 1998, Mahwah, NJ: Lawrence Erlbaum Associates.

were at risk or concluded that because they were not as promiscuous as Johnson, they were not likely to contract HIV through unsafe sex.

His name notwithstanding, Johnson's announcement did not work magic. It neither shattered illusions of invulnerability nor led to long-term behavioral change. But the revelation seems to have initiated the change process, moving some individuals closer to contemplating changes in their risk-behavior habits, perhaps pushing them from precontemplation to the contemplation stage of behavioral change or encouraging them to view AIDS not as an ugly abstraction but as an authentic problem, a potentially personally relevant concern (Kalichman, 1994).

How can we explain the effects of Magic Johnson's disclosure? One theory emphasizes identification. According to this view, people change attitudes because they like or identify with the communicator. Individuals' emotional involvement with and perceived similarity to Magic Johnson pushed them to call hotlines and get tested (e.g., Brown & Basil, 1995; Kelman, 1958). The contrast between Johnson's clean-cut, handsome image and the unpleasant ghoulish stereotype of AIDS made his announcement all the more cognitively memorable or accessible in memory.

Magic Johnson's disclosure also influenced attitudes toward individuals with HIV/AIDS. Prior to Johnson's announcement, public opinion toward people suffering from HIV was dominated by ugly abstractions, such as stereotypes of homosexuals or negative images of Rock Hudson (Pryor & Reeder, 1993). But Johnson changed this, providing people with a clean-cut, positive image of a person with HIV. One study found that the percentage of men who volunteered to help a person living with AIDS increased significantly following Johnson's announcement (Penner & Fritzsche, 1993). On a larger, societal level, Magic Johnson's disclosure may have transformed public perceptions of AIDS, bringing a sensitive topic into mainstream public discussion and encouraging people to perceive AIDS less as a problem of "them"—marginalized social groups— and more one to be faced by "all of us" (Moskowitz et al., 1997).

A decade has passed since Johnson revealed his condition. He is currently active in AIDS prevention campaigns and continues to be a positive role model. Johnson makes an excellent physical impression. His physical appeal enhances his persuasiveness, but may also have a more disturbing impact. Many men do not have money to purchase protease inhibitor drugs that reduce the ravages of HIV infection, nor can they afford the lifestyle that permits cultivation of a handsome physique. Johnson's ability to stay and look healthy, despite contracting HIV, may suggest to some people that they can engage in as much unsafe sex as they want because if Magic can lick HIV, then so can they. Unfortunately, not everyone will be so lucky.

MESSAGE CHARACTERISTICS

Fear Appeals

AIDS is scary. It scares the daylights out of people. Should communicators appeal to people's fears in an effort to increase AIDS prevention behaviors? And if so, how should they design the message?

These questions strike to the heart of research on fear appeals, a classic area in the psychology of persuasive communication. **A fear appeal is a persuasive communication that tries to scare people into changing their attitudes by conjuring up negative consequences that will occur if they do not comply with the message recommendations.** Fear messages typically appeal to individuals' self-interest to protect themselves against unwanted danger. Thus, much of the theorizing about fear appeals is consistent with the cognitive decision approaches discussed in this book, particularly the health belief model, which assumes that people make decisions based on their appraisal of the personal costs and benefits of health recommendations.

Some people believe that fear appeals work. Others say that individuals panic when they hear messages that try to scare them into changing a valued behavior. When faced with disagreements about the likely effects of persuasive communications, it is best to turn to theory and research.

The most comprehensive theory of fear appeals to date has been proposed by Kim Witte (1992, 1998). Called the **extended parallel process model,** the model extends previous research on fear appeals (e.g., Rogers, 1975) in key ways. The model also invokes *parallel processes* that have important but distinctive psychological effects on appraisals of fear messages. Although the model's components are complicated, the underlying thesis is delightfully simple. As Witte (1997) notes:

> Fear appeals are extremely effective persuasive strategies—but only under certain conditions. . . . After you scare someone about terrible outcomes and make them feel vulnerable to negative consequences, you must tell them clearly and explicitly how to prevent this outcome from occurring. . . . If a campaign only succeeds in scaring its audience or in increasing perceived vulnerability, it will fail (according to prevailing research). The reason it will fail is that the campaign only persuaded people to fear a health threat or consequence, but didn't teach them how to prevent it. (p. 151)

Let's now look at the model more carefully. Like other theorists, Witte (1998) distinguishes between fear, an internal emotional reaction, and threat, a danger that resides in the external environment. Arguing that you need to do more than scare people to change attitudes, Witte emphasizes that health communication messages should contain both a *threat* component and an *efficacy* component. The threat component is negative: It provides people with unpleasant

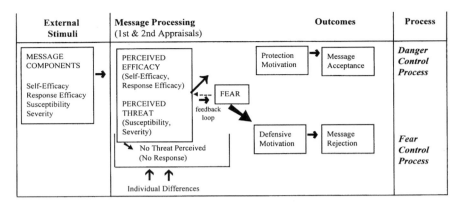

FIG. 5.4.   The Extended Parallel Process Model. From "Fear as motivator, fear as inhibitor: Using the extended parallel process model to explain fear appeal successes and failures" (p. 432), by K. Witte. In P. A. Andersen and L. K. Guerrero (Eds.), *Handbook of Communication and Emotion: Research, Theory, Applications, and Contexts*, 1998, San Diego, CA: Academic Press.

facts designed to scare them. The efficacy component is positive. It suggests what people can do to avert the threat.

More specifically, the threat portion of the message tries to convince individuals that they are *susceptible* to a *severe* threat. The efficacy portion attempts to persuade them that the recommended response effectively deters the threat (*response efficacy*), and that they are capable of performing the recommended response (*self-efficacy*). Note that the model draws on other theories I have discussed, notably the Health Belief Model and social cognitive theory (see Fig. 5.4).

According to the model, individuals first judge the severity of the threat and their susceptibility to it. If they view the threat as trivial or irrelevant, they proceed no further, sensing there is little reason to attend to the message.

However, if the threat is seen as severe and relevant to the self, people become frightened and motivated to take action (Witte et al., 1998). This is a critical moment in the time line of message processing as the fear evoked by the message can lead to one of two responses. People may decide that they can *control the danger* and successfully cope. Alternatively, they may panic and decide the threat is too scary and coping is beyond them. When this happens, people focus on the fear itself, trying to reduce their anxiety and engaging in a process of *fear control*.

What determines whether people will cope effectively—and deal with the external danger—or ineffectively, in which case they obsess on the internal fear? *A major factor is whether the communication persuades people that they are capable of performing an effective coping response.* If individuals feel capable of performing an effective recommended action, their feelings of efficacy will outweigh feelings of fear, and they will take steps to protect themselves.

By contrast, if perceived threat exceeds perceived efficacy, people shift into fear control mode. Witte (1998) notes that "people engage in fear control processes when they do not think they are able to adopt an effective response to avert a serious and relevant threat because the response is too hard, too costly, takes too much time, or they think it will not work" (p. 430). If a fear-arousing appeal elicits defensive or avoidance responses, the person rejects the message.

Why Safer Sex Appeals Fail. Witte's model helps us understand why AIDS fear messages frequently fail. Some messages don't get to first base because they are too hokey or far-fetched to arouse fear. For example, consider this safer sex message that appeared in an Ann Landers column:

> I want you young men to realize that for 10 to 15 minutes of unprotected sex, you could be paying 17 percent of your salary for the next 21 years to support the baby you just made. And pray the girl doesn't have twins . . . And now I would like to tell you young women that for 10 to 15 minutes of unprotected sex you may have to pay a lawyer thousands of dollars to try and collect child support. (Landers, 1998, p. 29)

These arguments are not credible to young people. The message tries to scare people by raising the specter of terrible consequences down the road. But teenagers reading this column would have trouble processing these consequences because they don't think down the road. Teens typically think they will live forever and they have trouble imagining bad outcomes that might occur when they grow up.

Other fear appeals fail for a different reason: They arouse too much anxiety, driving individuals into fear control mode. A case in point is news media coverage during the 1980s of heterosexuals' susceptibility to HIV infection.

Reacting to medical authorities' statements about the threat of heterosexual AIDS and (it must be said) eager to cover a dramatic, sensational story, the news media jumped on the heterosexual AIDS bandwagon in the late 1980s. Story after story suggested that American young people who practiced unsafe sex were highly susceptible to a severe threat: HIV infection.

A February 1987 *Time* article announced "The Big Chill: Fear of AIDS." The article dramatized the threat of heterosexual AIDS with "moralistic quotations . . . descriptions of heterosexuals who contracted AIDS after relatively few sexual encounters," and discussion of the "potential unreliability of condoms" (Brenders & Garrett, 1993, pp. 121–122). An *Atlantic Monthly* article published the same month emphasized heterosexuals' vulnerability without calling attention to ways of coping with the problem (Brenders & Garrett, 1993). The crowning moment of media hype came on February 18, 1987 when Oprah Winfrey claimed that "one in five heterosexuals could be dead from AIDS at the end of the next 3 years." The doomsday projections turned out to be wildly exaggerated. Although HIV infection among young people has increased in recent years and heterosexuals who engage in risky sex with multiple partners do increase their chances of contracting the virus, there is no AIDS epidemic among American heterosexual young people and none is likely to emerge (Fumento, 1990).

To be sure, news media coverage performed a valuable service by informing heterosexual young people that they could be susceptible to a deadly disease. However, many stories provided more threatening than efficacious information, perhaps causing some members of the audience to feel there was little they could do to avert the threat. Feeling scared and overwhelmed, individuals moved into fear control mode, defensively avoiding information that might help them cope with the problem (Morris & Swann, 1996; Wiebe & Black, 1997). Rather than trying to control the danger, these folks denied it, revealing illusions of invulnerability. It seems likely that the media coverage left some individuals with a generalized anxiety that contained elements of realistic fear and dysfunctional helplessness. This was aptly expressed by a young writer who articulated the feelings of many of her peers:

> Heterosexuals are receiving vague signals. We're told that if we are sufficiently vigilant, we will probably be all right. We're being told to assume the worst and to not invite disaster by hoping for the best. We're being encouraged to keep our fantasies on a tight rein, otherwise we'll lose control of the whole buggy, and no one can say we weren't warned. So for us AIDS remains a private hell, smoldering beneath intimate conversations among friends and surfacing on those occasional sleepless nights when it occurs to us to wonder about it, upon which that dark hysterias sets in, and those catalogues of whom we've done it with and whom they might have done it with and oh-my-God-I'll-surely-die seem to project themselves onto the ceiling, the way fanged monsters did when we were children. But we fall asleep and then we wake up. And nothing has changed except our willingness to forget about it, which has become the ultimate survival mechanism. What my peers and I are left with is a generalized anxiety, a low-grade fear and anger that resides at the core of everything we do. Our attitudes have been affected by the disease by leaving us scared, but our behavior has stayed largely the same. One result is a corrosion of the soul, a chronic dishonesty and fear that will most likely damage us more than the disease itself. In this world, peace of mind is a utopian concept. (Daum, 1996, p. 33)

How Safer Sex Appeals Can Succeed.   Fear appeals are dicey weapons. Arouse too little fear and you fail to motivate individuals to take preventive action. Evoke too much fear and you push the denial button. As Kathryn Morris and William Swann (1996) observe, "The creators of AIDS-prevention programs must learn to walk the whisker-thin line between too little and too much—between making targets of persuasive communications care enough to attend to the message but not dismiss the message through denial processes" (p. 70). Theory and research on the psychology of fear suggest several strategies for safer sex message design.

1. *Communications must "get 'em sick and then get 'em well."* After scaring individuals by telling them they are susceptible to a severe threat, persuasion campaigns must leave individuals with hope that if they adopt the recommended action, they can effectively cope with the problematic behavior. Fear appeals must teach, as well as scare. They must also impart the message clearly and explicitly.

2. *Media fear appeals should be of high production quality.* Although people do not like to admit that they are susceptible to persuasion, they are comfortable acknowledging that high-quality AIDS public service ads influence them personally (Duck, Terry, & Hogg, 1995). When ads are clever and evoke an emotional response, it reflects positively on the self to admit that you have been influenced. The only way that communications can shatter the illusion of invulnerability is to convey information so persuasively that it would be embarrassing not to admit that the messages make a good point.

3. *Efficacy recommendations should emphasize costs of not taking precautionary action as well as benefits of undertaking the activity.* Research based on information-processing theory suggests that communications will be more effective if they emphasize what people lose from *not* practicing safer sex or *not* getting tested for HIV rather than the benefits of these activities (Kalichman & Coley, 1995). Thus, campaigns would be better advised to vividly describe case studies of individuals who failed to employ condoms and contracted a sexually transmitted disease than to focus on people who always negotiate condom use successfully (Thompson et al., 1999).

4. *AIDS threats and recommendations should be salient—or relevant—to the target audience.* Campaign practitioners cannot assume that what scares them also scares their target audience. Furthermore, different fears will be salient to different groups. As the last chapter indicated, a poor woman of color may be more scared about losing her man than getting an STD. However, a fear appeal that broaches this too directly will push the woman into denial. A successful fear appeal will walk the razor-thin line between getting the woman to care enough to pay attention to the message, but not dismiss the message through denial.

Accommodation Versus Confrontation

When designing HIV prevention messages, should you accommodate audience members, trying to understand their concerns and matching your message to their needs? Or should you try to shake people up, make them uncomfortable, and use the discomfort you arouse to propel them toward attitude change? Research on fear appeals suggests you should do a little of both.

More generally, three persuasion theories urge accommodation and one prominent theory recommends confrontation. Because both accommodation and confrontation are useful strategies, it is helpful to review the implications of these theories for AIDS prevention behavior. I begin with theories that fall under an accommodation label: the **theory of reasoned action (TRA); elaboration likelihood model (ELM), and speech accommodation theory.**

Theory of Reasoned Action. As discussed in chapter 2, the TRA emphasizes that persuaders cannot change AIDS-related attitudes unless they tap into salient or relevant concerns of the audience. Stipulating that attitude and subjective norm determine behavioral intention and intentions predict behavior under most circumstances, the theory identifies five factors that can be the focus of communication interventions. They are: (a) beliefs about a particular behavior, (b) evaluations of these beliefs, (c) beliefs that important others recommend performance of the behavior, (d) motivation to comply with these significant others, and (e) behavioral intention.

Theorists emphasize that persuaders should focus an intervention on a highly specific behavior. For example, a campaign might be planned to strengthen young women's intention to purchase latex condoms at a campus drugstore (Wilson et al., 1993). Practitioners would want to first identify the salient behavioral and normative beliefs of the target audience. Marketing research might tell us that women: (a) believe that purchasing a condom at the local drugstore would suggest they are "loose" and "available for sex," (b) feel negatively toward loose available women, (c) perceive that close friends attach a stigma to women buying condoms at a campus drugstore, (d) feel impelled to follow their friends' recommendations, and (e) therefore don't intend to buy condoms at the drugstore.

Practitioners could direct communications at any of these constructs. They would decide which element to target based on survey research. Persuaders might opt to counteract behavioral beliefs, perhaps by suggesting that purchasing condoms is a good way to show self-respect and respect for one's partner. This would help change the meaning that young women attribute to condom purchases. Messages might alter subjective norms by providing authentic comments from female undergraduates who regularly buy condoms at a drugstore and don't find them stigmatizing. Humor could also be used to deflect negative attitudes.

Elaboration Likelihood Model. The ELM gears the message to people's strategy for processing messages. The model says that people process persuasive messages either centrally or peripherally (Petty, Gleicher, & Jarvis, 1993). When people process information centrally (through *a central route*), they think a great deal, assess the quality of message arguments, and draw on previous experiences. Central processing is careful and systematic. It assumes that the person is motivated and able to think about the message. Since the individual expends a lot of energy thinking about the communication, attitudes formed via central route processing tend to be well integrated into the person's belief system. Consequently, these attitudes persist for a long time.

In other cases, people take the easy way out, processing information superficially or through *a peripheral route*. When people process information peripherally, they rely on mental shortcuts and simple cues, such as whether the source is an expert. When people don't care about an issue or perceive they are low in ability, they take the peripheral route. For example, people frequently lack time or motivation to think deeply about which gum, paper towel, or soft drink to buy. Recognizing this, advertisers rely on numerous peripheral cues to promote these products, including humor, celebrity endorsements, and glitzy packaging.

According to the ELM, a key element in persuasion is matching the message to the motivation (or involvement) level of the person. You would not want to send a superficial message to a person deeply concerned about an issue. They'd be insulted. Conversely, you wouldn't want to deliver a complex, intellectual communication to someone who is uninterested in the topic. They'd fall asleep.

The model has interesting implications for AIDS prevention persuasion. If an individual is concerned about HIV infection—that is, highly motivated to process the message—the persuader should prepare a communication that gets the person thinking or ties in with deep-seated values. Unfortunately, the ELM does not tell us just how to devise these messages. Happily, the model provides more clues on how to reach less-motivated—low-involved—message receivers.

Reaching those with little apparent interest in safer sex issues is important because such individuals may be at risk for AIDS but be unwilling to think about it. Here is where celebrity spokespersons, like Magic Johnson, can play an important role. Low-involved individuals, lacking motivation to carefully think about what the communicator says, may adopt message recommendations simply because the messenger is famous or has that celebrity "glow." Simple, visual safer sex messages have also proven to be effective with individuals who do not enjoy thinking or expending energy on cognitive tasks (Bakker, 1999).

According to the ELM, the best way to reach low-involved, at-risk individuals is not to hit them over the head with a strong fear appeal or force-feed them thought-provoking arguments about HIV infection. Instead, persuaders should start small, captivating them with simple appeals and, as they become more involved in HIV prevention, gradually upgrade the level of persuasive arguments.

Speech Accommodation Theory. Another approach that emphasizes accommodation is appropriately called speech accommodation theory (Giles & Smith, 1979). Although not a theory in the formal sense, speech accommodation formulates hypotheses and has implications for safer sex persuasion. According to speech accommodation theory, speakers gain favorable evaluations from listeners when they match their speech style to the listener. If most target audience members speak slowly and with an ethnic dialect, the speaker should do the same to maximize perceptions of similarity and likability. For example, HIV prevention messages geared to inner-city African American youths should use language congenial with the "tell it like it is," antimainstream quality of current hip-hop culture (McLaurin, 1995).

By contrast, messages geared to educated middle-class parents should reflect the speech style of mainstream United States. A speaker who tries to use hip street talk in an effort to underscore the reality of HIV/AIDS may lose credibility with this audience. For example, a sex education expert recently spoke to parents of children at my son's elementary school. Trying to impress parents with his knowledge of youth sexuality, he used slang, obscenities, and street language. He also surprised parents by showing lewd pictures of sexual penetration. Even I, who recognize the need to educate parents about AIDS and write on these issues on a daily basis, was surprised by his approach. Other parents were taken aback—not by his message but by how he communicated it. His audience was parents of kindergarten to fifth graders, not parents of high school kids. Not only did he arouse fear that was inappropriate to parents of children of this age level without providing solutions, he also used coarse language that offended many parents.

Confronting the Audience

Is it ever appropriate to diverge from the audience? Should a persuader aim to confront audience members in an effort to persuade? In a word, yes.

According to *cognitive dissonance theory,* people are disturbed by inconsistencies between their thoughts and actions. Individuals are especially vexed when they do something that violates their view of themselves. Dissonance theory says that people experience discomfort when they perform a behavior that is inconsistent with an attitude or self-concept. One way to reduce dissonance is to change the attitude so it fits the behavior.

Suppose, knowing this, a persuader deliberately induces people to say something they don't believe. Dissonance theory suggests that having engaged in the counterattitudinal behavior, people will feel motivated to change their attitude in the direction of the behavior they just performed. This can be applied rather neatly to AIDS preventive attitudes, as Jeff Stone and his colleagues (1994) demonstrated. The authors noted that:

> Our application of dissonance and self-persuasion to the prevention of AIDS takes advantage of an existing hypocrisy—the fact that most college students believe they should systematically use condoms to prevent AIDS but do not always behave according to this belief. . . . Suppose subjects are then made mindful of the fact that they themselves do not use condoms regularly; the resulting inconsistency between their public commitment and the increased awareness of their current risky sexual behavior should cause dissonance. To reduce dissonance, subjects are expected to begin to practice what they preach—that is, to change their sexual behavior, effectively bringing their practice of safe sex in line

with their preachings about the importance of condom use for AIDS prevention. (p. 117)

In a nifty experiment, Stone and his colleagues proved their point. Participants in the study were led to believe they were helping design an AIDS prevention program to be used at the high school level. Experimental group subjects wrote a persuasive speech about safer sex and delivered it in front of a video camera. Some subjects read about circumstances that made it difficult for people to use condoms. They also made a list of reasons why they had not used condoms in the past. This was designed to arouse cognitive dissonance—that is, induce feelings of hypocrisy in the students. (Control group subjects did not list these reasons or did not make the safer sex speech before a video camera.) All students were given an opportunity to buy condoms, using the $4 they had earned for participating in the experiment.

As predicted, more subjects in the hypocrisy condition purchased condoms and bought more condoms than students in control conditions. Their behavior was apparently motivated by the discomfort they experienced when they recognized that they do not always practice what they preach.

As interesting as the findings are, caution is needed when suggesting that hypocrisy induction is a panacea for safer sex persuasion. Subjects faced none of the pressures to engage in unsafe sex that afflict people in the real world. As chapters 3 and 4 described, these pressures include a desire to maintain intimacy, fear of offending a partner, and even anxiety about being physically assaulted if one proposes condom use. Nonetheless, hypocrisy induction—provided it does not make people feel defensive about their incongruent behavior—is a novel way to encourage people to practice safer sex. Ironically, this confrontational strategy must be applied gingerly, with consideration for the social context in which the intervention takes place.

Summary. In the final analysis, both accommodation and confrontation are useful in AIDS prevention campaigns. If persuaders do not accommodate the target audience, they will not reach them psychologically; the audience will tune out the message. But if communicators worry so much about pleasing individuals that they don't tell them painful truths, people will lack motivation to change. Hypocrisy induction, if used properly, can motivate individuals to change AIDS-related attitudes. For example, one can imagine trying to remind HIV-positive gay men who are tempted to manipulate other men into unprotected sex of their long-held commitment to gay liberation and empowerment. One can envision trying to persuade single Latina mothers not to choose unsafe sex by reminding them what would happen to their families—and their commitment to being good mothers—if they became infected with HIV. Gently confronting people while showing empathy to their needs, combining confrontation with accommodation, is a potentially effective way to begin the process of AIDS prevention change.

BEHAVIORAL SKILLS TRAINING

• It's a Friday night, and Monique is sitting in the car with her date. They've been necking a little, but now he's getting more serious. She likes his company but doesn't want to have sex with him. Through his words and actions she can tell he's pushing to have sex. He says: "Oh, come on. We know each other well, so let's do it."

• Susan is alone and homeless. She lives in shelters, but because they must limit her stay to 30 days, she often finds herself on the streets with nowhere to stay. At those times, Susan hangs out with others who drink and often ends up sleeping on the floor of any member of the group who has an apartment. Sex is often the price for a place to stay.

• Mark is 16 and was kicked out of the home of his mother and stepfather after frequent and violent conflicts. He now lives on the streets in a large city. Mark's life is in turmoil as he and a large number of other homeless or runaway teenagers shift about finding places to stay and eat and ways to make money. Sometimes Mark does odd jobs. But, Mark has also learned that he can hustle sex to older men for money. You can make more by having sex without a condom than with one. (adapted from Kelly, 1995, pp. 107, 126)

These vignettes illustrate the challenges of negotiating safer sex. Source and message strategies can persuade individuals like Monique, Susan, and Mark that they are at risk and need to change dysfunctional behaviors. However, standard persuasion approaches do not go far enough. Campaigns must not only convince people they are at risk but also teach them to perform behaviors that will ward off the danger. Cognitive-behavior models, such as Bandura's self-efficacy approach, planned behavior theory, and the array of interpersonal communication approaches discussed in chapter 3, offer suggestions for how to help individuals develop self-management and sexual communication skills. This section draws on the pioneering work of Jeffrey Fisher and William Fisher, and Jeffrey Kelly.

Information–Motivation–Behavioral Skills (IMB) Model

The IMB model identifies three important components of AIDS behavior change: information, motivation, and behavioral skills. The model links the components together in a coherent fashion (see Fig. 5.5).

Information and motivation are regarded as independent entities. "Well-informed individuals may have either high or low motivation to practice AIDS-preventive behavior," Fisher and Fisher (1996) note, "and well-motivated individuals may or may not be well informed" (p. 104).

Information is the first critical step in the IMB approach. Information is important because people cannot enact AIDS preventive behavior if they do not

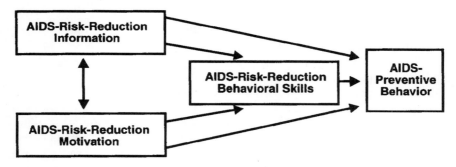

FIG. 5.5.   The Information–Motivation–Behavioral Skills (IMB) Model.

know how AIDS is transmitted or can be prevented. As we have seen, people can be woefully misinformed about AIDS transmission routes. For example, about one third of a sample of adolescent mothers—some of whom were probably involved with injecting drug users—did not know that sexual partners of IDUs are at risk to get AIDS (Brown et al., 1998). In Thailand, some young women incorrectly believe that HIV is transmitted by mosquitoes, toilets, and air conditioners. According to the IMB, information is needed to correct misperceptions. However, knowledge is not enough. Research indicates that people can be highly informed about HIV transmission but still engage in risky behavior (e.g., Díaz, 1998; Sheeran et al., 1999; Sobo, 1995). This is because they can know how the disease is spread but not believe that this knowledge applies to them personally, or lack adequate motivation to put knowledge into practice.

Motivation, the second component of the IMB, refers to attitudes toward AIDS precautionary behaviors and perceived social support for performing such acts. The model stipulates that individuals must be highly motivated to initiate and sustain AIDS behavioral changes.

The core component of the model is behavioral skills. According to the IMB, information about AIDS risk reduction and motivation activates behavioral skills, such as the ability to communicate about safer sex issues with one's partner. Armed with these skills, people are better able to sustain long-term behavioral change.

The IMB has been employed programmatically to change AIDS risk-reduction information, motivation, and behavior. A key tenet of the model is that interventions must be tailored to the targeted population. Pilot research is conducted to identify the particular deficits in information, motivation, and behavioral skills that are unique to the group the campaigner is trying to reach. Armed with this information, practitioners mount elaborate interventions and assess their effects. The interventions, frequently conducted with university students, have been very successful and are described in the next chapter.

A COGNITIVE, COMMUNICATION APPROACH
TO BEHAVIORAL SKILLS TRAINING

Another approach to teaching AIDS preventive skills is derived from social cognitive theory. In his work on this subject, Bandura (1990, 1994) argues that campaigns must do four things: (a) provide information to increase awareness of HIV risk, (b) teach self-management and sexual communication skills, (c) strengthen perceived self-efficacy, and (d) create social support and reinforcement for efforts to modify problematic behaviors. A social cognitive approach emphasizes that skills training is a step-by-step process involving modeling of behavior by trusted others, cognitive rehearsal of the modeled behavior, self-efficacy instruction, reinforcement and feedback to correct dysfunctional responses, and continued practice until the behavior has become an accepted part of the person's repertoire.

All well and good. But in the area of safer sex, words do not translate easily into deeds. Kelly (1995) identifies three barriers that can impede implementation of safer sex behavior change:

1. The behavior changes needed to curtail risk are less rewarding, more awkward, and more difficult than unsafe sex.
2. Behavior change efforts often meet with resistance from sexual partners.
3. Even persons who are at great risk rarely seek out behavior-change assistance. (pp. 17, 96)

Fortunately, there are ways to help people change dysfunctional risk reduction behaviors. Some observers argue that the best prevention is to engage in the safest sex of all: abstinence or sexual practices other than vaginal or anal intercourse. This is certainly a laudable goal, particularly with teenagers. The problem, metaphorically speaking, is that it is tough to convince people to turn down the heat when they've made unprotected love in the kitchen. Many people don't want to abstain from sexual intercourse. It is, therefore, more reasonable to gear interventions toward increasing condom use, particularly by enhancing sexual communication skills.

How do campaign practitioners teach individuals—persuade them, perhaps —to change intimate sexual behaviors? How do they help them develop skills needed to avoid risky situations? Let's look at several key areas, drawing on social cognitive theory and interpersonal communication concepts.

Increasing Skill in Using Condoms

Increase ability to put on condoms? Come on, it's not brain surgery, right? Surprising as it seems, some people don't know how to use condoms competently, harbor misconceptions about condoms, or are so eager to have sex that they ignore common sense. As one family planning expert related, "If you're talking about adolescents who are frustrated or nervous, they just give up because they don't want their partner to know that they don't know how to put a condom on" (Snowbeck, 1999, p. F-1).

Consider that some people harbor mistaken beliefs about condoms; they think that condoms can be reused (Not!) and that all condoms are equal (Wrong: Latex condoms are better because HIV can seep through nonlatex models). Laraine Winter and Susan Goldy (1993) devised an intervention to promote condom use. They gave subjects experience handling a condom, opening the package, and rolling the condom over their fingers. They found that experience combined with role-playing on how to deal with partner reservations about condom use increased condom acceptance.

Disassociating Alcohol Use From Sex

"Just because you see people putting condoms in their pockets, it doesn't mean they are using them," a student recently told a pollster. "If you meet someone at a bar and there is alcohol involved, then communication can go out the window," the student added (MacDonald, Zanna, & Fong, 1996, p. 763).

Research backs up this supposition (Gordon, Carey, & Carey, 1997; MacDonald et al., 1996). Four studies conducted by Tara MacDonald and her colleagues (1996) found that alcohol reduces the likelihood of condom use during casual sexual intercourse. As the researchers remind us, when people are drunk, they have trouble taking a long-term perspective; instead, they focus on the most salient, exciting aspects of the situation. Sex trumps rational processing. Obviously, the best thing to do is to convince people to stop drinking or quit having so much sex. However, these are difficult objectives because both drinking and sex fulfill important psychological needs.

How do you encourage individuals who enjoy worldly pleasures to disassociate alcohol from risky sex? A behavioral skills approach suggests that persuasive communicators should start by providing information. For example, a public service announcement (PSA) could let audiences know that people have difficulty refusing unprotected sex when they are drunk. Using dramatic devices, the PSA could provide counterarguments that audience members could use if they ever found themselves in this situation (MacDonald et al., 1996). Another strategy is to help people disassociate drinking and sex by encouraging them to think of "times for drinking" as different than "times for sexual intimacy" so that the two activities do not overlap so much (Kelly, 1995).

Changing Negative Attitudes Toward Condom Use

As noted in chapter 2, beliefs about condoms and negative evaluations of these beliefs underlie unfavorable attitudes toward safer sex. Although changing attitudes is never easy, Kelly suggests chipping away at negative condom attitudes by reframing beliefs and countering perceived disadvantages of condoms with perceived benefits. Consider four negative attitudes people have toward condoms and ways of countering them:

Negative Attitude	Relabeled Statement
Condom use implies a lack of trust.	Using condoms is the best way to show someone that you care about them.
Using condoms is awkward and interrupts sex.	Condom use is fun when it becomes a part of sex and love-making.
Condoms reduce pleasure.	Condoms can increase pleasure by reducing worries about sex and pregnancy.
Condoms imply that you are dirty.	Condoms make sex healthier and clean, and they show you are proud of yourself. (Kelly, 1995, p. 99)

One aim of these efforts is to eroticize safer sex. Despite the laudable objective, efforts to associate condoms with sexuality are not going to work for everyone, particularly those who have sexual inhibitions or oppose condoms on religious grounds. Conversely, people who get great satisfaction from unprotected sexual pleasure may never find condoms "fun." However, many others are open to gentle persuasion. Cognitive theory suggests that for these individuals, condom discussion should be reframed in the ways suggested above. The goal is to make condom use so common that it becomes an accepted part of young people's sexual scripts, one that comes automatically to mind when sex begins "heating up." As one family planning expert put it, "You have to make it so hip to use a condom that people almost would be ashamed not to use it" (Snowbeck, 1999, p. F-2).

Communication and Compliance

Communication plays a critical role in safer sex persuasion. Couples who can talk openly about health and condom use are more likely to practice safer sex than couples who do not discuss these issues (Catania et al., 1992). Communication is particularly important for women, as Judith Goldman and Lisa Harlow (1993) explain:

> In order for condom use to occur, a woman may have to insist that the man put on a condom, whereas a man merely needs to make the decision to wear one. In effect, the woman in this situation has less control than the man. Her preventive behavior seems to be less dependent on her own internal feelings and more dependent on her communication skills. (p. 495)

How can practitioners teach people to communicate more skillfully about safer sex and AIDS prevention? Social psychological and interpersonal communication theories offer some clues. In a systematic investigation of safer sex compliance-gaining, Bradley Reel and Teresa Thompson (1994) reported that young people are more comfortable discussing condoms in terms of preventing pregnancy than HIV prevention. They also found that "all one needs to do is *bring up* the topic of AIDS or condoms in order to get a partner to use a condom" (p. 137). These findings provide reason for optimism and suggest that, at least among college students (the bulk of Reel and Thompson's sample), simply broaching the topic is enough. However, data reviewed in earlier chapters indicate that, although people tell researchers they intend to use a condom, they may resist condom use in actual situations. Intentions will not predict behaviors when people perceive they lack control over the behavior in question. Improved communication skills are particularly important for poor minority women who may harbor positive intentions toward condom use but be scared to translate intentions into action.

How do practitioners help people develop these skills? What strategies work best to gain safer sex compliance? There is no consensus at the present time. Some scholars say that partners should be up front and honest, whereas others correctly point out that an overly blunt approach—"While I like you, I'm not willing to die for you"—can backfire and lead to an argument (Kelly, 1995, p. 115; Reel & Thompson, 1994). Still other experts urge partners to avoid thinking of sex as negotiation, but rather as playful activity that can be made more enjoyable by seductive use of condoms (Adelman, 1992). One thing that researchers acknowledge is that compliance-gaining efforts must be tailored to a particular situation—that is, to the needs of a partner, the relationship, cultural setting, and the possibility that the request may meet with resistance.

For its part, interpersonal communication research emphasizes that condom-use communication is bound to be dynamic and characterized by both partners' attempts to maintain a positive impression, save face, and accomplish relational goals. Successful condom-use conversations will have to take these factors into account. What's more, individuals will be more likely to convince a partner to use a condom (or to engage in other AIDS precautionary behaviors) if they develop a specific *mental plan* beforehand (Waldron et al., 1995). Many people who meticulously plan their work day and important career moves enter sexual situations impulsively, with nary a plan nor idea of how to influence a partner's safer sex choices and what to do if he or she refuses.

Waldron's research suggests that people should develop a variety of specific plans to influence a partner to use a condom. Vague plans ("I'll just bring it up when we're making love") are less likely to be effective, perhaps because the individual has not thought through what to do if the partner objects.

Not all researchers believe that sex partners should spend their spare time thinking through safer sex contingency plans. Mara Adelman (1992) suggests that scholars should lighten up, remember that sex involves passion, and use more playful, spontaneous ways to encourage partners to practice safer sex (see Boxes 5.1 and 5.2). I believe there is room for both approaches. Playful, humorous approaches can deflect the tension and help partners reframe a stressful situation. At the same time, some people would prefer to practice safer sex and intend to bring this up with a partner, but chicken out at the last minute. For these individuals—perhaps teenagers or poor ethnic women—planning what to say beforehand can help them accomplish a personally important goal. Besides, it's hard to see how a plan could destroy the spontaneity and sheer pleasure of sex!

In addition to communication approaches, social psychological theories like Bandura's self-efficacy model can be helpful in designing AIDS prevention interventions. There are a variety of ways to increase self-efficacy, including modeling, reinforcement, cognitive rehearsal (Maibach & Flora, 1993), role-playing, and self-reinforcement (whereby people learn to praise themselves for making tough safer sex choices). It is especially important to help people access these skills when sex gets heated and the last thing they want to do is pick up a condom.

Building on these ideas, a generalized skills perspective suggests that communicators teach individuals the behavioral skills needed to get them to feel comfortable talking about safer sex, and the cognitive skills that will ensure they can carry out this task in difficult interpersonal situations. Kelly (1995) sums it up nicely:

> Different communication styles work best for different people, and it is important that the assertive approach taken—whether firmly direct, humorous, cajoling, sexual, or imbedded in the context of messages that affirm affection and caring for the partner to defuse negative reactions—be tailored to the relationship and the expected response of the partner. This does not mean that clients should back away from their safer sex insistence position. Instead, it means that flexibility in the style of assertiveness used is needed to maximize the likelihood that a partner will comply with the request. (p. 116)

CONCLUSION

This chapter has applied theories of persuasion to AIDS prevention behavior, notably safer sex. Changing behavior is not a simple process but a complex one that proceeds over a series of steps and unfolds over time. Models of behavior change, such as the AIDS Risk Reduction Model and the transtheoretical model, emphasize that individuals must first label their risky behavior as problematic, contemplate ways to change their behavior, plan to make a change in an attitude or action, and begin taking steps to change the risky behavior. McGuire's input–output model of persuasive communication suggests ways that communications can help individuals achieve these goals.

BOX 5.1

HUMOR AND SAFER SEX

Communication expert Mara Adelman (1992) suggests that practitioners could help people talk more comfortably about condom use if they used a little humor. View safer sex as play, she urges campaign planners and sexual partners. If you think of sex in this way, it could help people cope better with embarrassment and assist them in redefining a stressful situation. Here are two compliance-gaining dramatizations she created that could be useful in media campaigns. (In the scenes that follow, F refers to female; M to male.)

Message 1

F: Right, and I want to think about using a . . .

M: One of those.

F: I really do.

M: A . . . a raincoat [smiling up at her]. Is that what you're driving at?

F: Yes, a glove.

M: [laughing] I have one of those [they kiss, then the male looking mischievously at the female]. I have a whole box of them.

F: You do?

M: Pristine, unopened box [kiss]. We could use [kiss] every single one of them.

Message 2

F: Well, actually I'm on the pill. But if you don't mind I'd like to take some precaution.

M: Double protection. Aquafresh [reference to a toothpaste commercial].

F: The pill doesn't protect against everything . . . It's not like I don't trust you.

M: I understand that, but you don't have to worry, because it's not a problem.

F: Thanks.

M: I also have these condoms that a friend of mine sent me from Tijuana that have those Goodyear radial ribs on them that will drive you wild.

F: [loud laughter]

M: If you want, I don't have to drive you wild, we can have a more sedate evening.

F: No, wildness would be fine.

From Adelman (1992), p. 82.

BOX 5.2

IF COMPANIES ADVERTISED CONDOMS . . .

A little humor can go a long way toward deflecting tension surrounding AIDS and safer sex. Take, for example, the following campaign ideas that appeared on a web site:

Nike Condoms: Just do it.

Toyota Condoms: Oh, what a feeling.

Diet Pepsi Condoms: You got the right one, baby.

Pringles Condoms: Once you pop, you can't stop.

Chevy Condoms: Like a rock.

Dial Condoms: Aren't you glad you use it? Don't you wish everybody did?

Avis Condoms: Trying harder than ever.

Lays Condoms: Betcha can't have just one.

Campbell's Soup Condoms: Mmm, mmm, good.

AT&T Condoms: Reach out and touch someone.

Bounty Condoms: The quicker picker upper.

M&M Condoms: It melts in your mouth, not in your hands!

Delta Airlines travel pack Condoms: Delta is ready when you are.

Star Trek Condoms: To Boldly Go Where No Man Has Gone Before.

From "So which condom would you use . . .? (1998). This list was found at http://www.msu.edu/user/bangjaem/text/condom.htm but is no longer available online.

Source approaches stress that communicators who are perceived as credible and similar to the recipient can change safer sex attitudes. Magic Johnson is a case in point. As an attractive, celebrity basketball player, his disclosure that he was HIV-positive was an immediate media event. Johnson's revelation spurred millions to call the National AIDS Hotline, increased concern about AIDS (particularly among African American men), and changed perceptions of AIDS from a marginalized disease to one that can potentially affect us all. The Johnson episode has important implications for AIDS prevention campaigns. Practitioners should prepare "generic intervention packages" in advance to take maximum advantage of the positive effects celebrity disclosures produce (Kalichman, 1994, p. 555).

Messages can also be geared to change safer sex perceptions and attitudes. Fear appeals can be very useful persuasive strategies, but only if certain conditions are met. Witte's model emphasizes that fear communications must contain a threat and efficacy component—that is, they must threaten people that bad things will happen if they don't change their behavior and also teach them how to prevent these threats from materializing. Some safer sex appeals failed because they did not scare the audience; the threats were too hokey or far-fetched. Others backfired for the opposite reason: They scared the audience too much, neglecting to tell people how to cope with the threat. Current research suggests ways that practitioners can design fear appeals so that they arouse appropriate doses of fear while also providing people with the tools to change behavior.

Other message approaches emphasize that communications can either accommodate or confront the audience. Accommodationist approaches include the theory of reasoned action, with its emphasis on tapping into salient or relevant audience concerns, the elaboration likelihood model, which says persuaders must match messages to the audience's level of involvement in AIDS prevention, and speech accommodation theory, which suggests that communicators use language that message receivers can relate to. Alternatively, persuaders can try to shake the audience up, showing them that they do not practice what they preach about safer sex. Hypocrisy induction, developed from cognitive dissonance theory, is an example of this. Needless to say, it must be used carefully, in a way that shows respect for individuals' needs.

Campaigns must not only change safer sex attitudes. They should also teach people risk-reduction behavioral skills that they can use in everyday situations. Fisher and Fisher's information-motivation-behavior model, Kelly's principles of behavioral skills acquisition, Bandura's self-efficacy approach, and communication approaches to safer sex compliance-gaining are all designed to enhance skills in safer sex self-management and negotiation.

None of these persuasion approaches work miracles. They all run up against psychological barriers, such as the pleasures unsafe sex offers people, anxieties about change, and fear of losing a valued relationship. Nonetheless, research suggests that these approaches can help people change attitudes. Most of all, they deliver the goods that theories are supposed to transport: ideas and new ways to help solve human problems.

CHAPTER SIX

AIDS Prevention Campaigns

A public service announcement depicts a couple in bed. They're giggling and play-ing footsie. The woman asks her lover if he has the condom. No—he's forgotten it. She reminds him that they had agreed to use one and says emphatically, "No condom, no sex." He rolls away from her, apparently annoyed, but the excitement is recaptured when he says he's going to make a trip to the late-night drugstore.

A second ad depicts a young couple about to go to bed. The bed is strewn with upright syringes. The narrator intones, "Before you go to bed with someone, ask yourself, Who have they been to bed with? They could have slept with someone who's been doing drugs and has shared a needle with someone who's had the AIDS virus. If you go to bed with someone, always use a condom, because when you sleep with someone, you're sleeping with their past." (Duck et al., 1995, pp. 311–312)

What do you think? Are these PSAs compelling? Hokey? Possibly effective? Whatever your reactions, you are no doubt familiar with AIDS public service announcements like these. They are part of the communication landscape in the United States and abroad, a familiar aspect of media campaigns. This chap-ter examines the structure and effects of such media and community-level AIDS prevention campaigns. It extends the exploration of AIDS, safer sex, and per-suasion to a larger macro level. Thus far, the predominant emphasis has been micro as I have examined ways in which messages influence beliefs and how people persuade themselves to modify risky sexual behaviors. However, in a large diversified society it is also necessary to harness community resources and devise mass media campaigns to reach individuals at risk for HIV infection and help them move through stages of change. This chapter discusses such macro-level communication interventions, applying knowledge of communication channels and receivers (based on McGuire's input–output matrix), as well as theories of social change. The chapter discusses how large-scale AIDS preven-tion campaigns are conducted, focuses on campaign limits and effects, and sug-gests how communication can be used to influence individuals in diverse AIDS risk groups. One of the themes of the chapter is that effective AIDS interven-tions require systematic application of theory, in-depth understanding of the target population, and keen use of community resources.

The first portion of this chapter reviews two theories that bear on the channel by which messages are communicated to the public. The second section examines how campaigns can be tailored to influence different at-risk groups. Using McGuire's scheme, the first section looks at channel factors, the second at receiver factors.

COMMUNICATION CHANNELS AND AIDS PREVENTION

Diffusion of Innovations

Everett Rogers (1995) developed and tested a theory of how innovations spread — or diffuse — through a society. His theory helps explain how change occurs and why certain changes occur faster than others. Communication is the centerpiece of diffusion of innovation theory. It is through communication that new ideas are diffused, adopted, or rejected. Many factors enter into the diffusion process, including characteristics of the innovation (e.g., its compatibility with existing values), communication channels (interpersonal and mass media), degree of innovativeness of members of a social system, and behavior of opinion leaders.

There has been considerable innovation in the area of AIDS prevention, and these innovations have diffused through society. Although condoms predate the discovery of the HIV, they were taboo topics until social change agents concluded that condoms could help prevent the spread of AIDS. Since the mid-1980s, condoms have become synonymous with HIV prevention. Their popularity has skyrocketed and it has become socially acceptable to talk about them in many public contexts, ranging from university classrooms to entertainment television shows. Although condom usage is sporadic among certain individuals and groups (as discussed in previous chapters), there is no doubt that millions of individuals world-wide know that condoms help prevent the spread of AIDS and that they *should* engage in safer sex. (Diffusion of the term *safer sex* also counts as an innovation.)

There have been other AIDS-related innovations, such as the use of bleach to disinfect HIV-contaminated needles. Politically, activist groups representing those who have contracted the virus (e.g., gay men) have organized to protest government indifference and to help community members develop safer health habits (Rogers et al., 1995). This is noteworthy when one considers that in other epidemics, victims (now a negatively charged word, also an innovation) passively accepted their fate (see Rushing, 1995, for a discussion of the plight of Jews during the Black Death and the poor during the 1830s cholera epidemic). Activist groups have innovatively opted to challenge the status quo, and health organizations have organized to provide AIDS-related services (San Francisco has more than 400 such groups), a development that was unthinkable in earlier epidemics.

From a persuasion point of view, the question is how AIDS prevention issues have been discussed in communication channels. Channels, defined as the modalities by which messages pass from one individual to another, include interpersonal communication, mass media, and combinations (e.g., Internet). According to diffusion theory, mass media are important in imparting knowledge of the innovation; interpersonal communication plays a vital role in helping to persuade people to change attitudes.

Mass Media.   In the United States, the media have exerted complex effects on knowledge about AIDS prevention and transmission. In some cases, the media have performed their jobs admirably, in other cases they have been laggards, resisting change. Early on, the news media shied away from covering the AIDS epidemic. Although people were dying from AIDS in the early 1980s, the story rarely made the front pages or evening news (Dearing & Rogers, 1992). Why?

One explanation is that journalists harbored an antigay prejudice that kept them from playing up the fact that many of those falling prey to the disease were sexually active gay men (Kinsella, 1988). Another factor, stemming from journalists' dependence on official sources, is that the Reagan White House did not regard AIDS as a major priority. Hence, few established sources talked about AIDS or leaked information to reporters. A third explanation is that AIDS deaths are slow and lingering, rather than fast-onset events like earthquakes and bombings that easily lend themselves to television coverage.

This changed in mid-1985, when Rock Hudson died of AIDS and controversy swirled over whether 13-year-old Ryan White, who had been diagnosed with HIV, should be permitted to attend school in Kokomo, Indiana. These events captured media interest. AIDS was no longer a "mysterious gay plague," but a disease that affected a world famous actor and school children in middle America (Dearing & Rogers, 1992). Two years later, as is typical with the press, the media did a 180-degree turn, covering the specter of (heterosexual) AIDS in great detail. In some instances the press served a valuable public health function, providing needed facts about HIV prevention. At other times, it sensationalized matters, as in the case of the heterosexual AIDS scare (see chapter 5). Since the 1980s, AIDS has become a regular staple in the press, gaining extensive coverage when a spectacular event happens (like Magic Johnson's announcement) or when a newspaper decides to do a feature on the HIV catastrophe in Africa. Alternative media, notably the gay press, have been replete with stories about AIDS and conflicts between gay activists and political authorities.

The entertainment media have focused on AIDS in spades. Occasionally, movies about AIDS make a big splash. An example is *Philadelphia,* in which Tom Hanks and Denzel Washington dramatically portrayed two lawyers who sue a law firm for AIDS discrimination. Numerous media documentaries about AIDS have been produced, and Internet sites are filled with AIDS information, ranging from news group dialogue to facts about HIV transmission.

Theory and research strongly suggest that the media greatly enhanced public knowledge of AIDS transmission. Because the media are the primary channel by which information about AIDS is diffused and AIDS knowledge levels have greatly increased over the course of the epidemic (e.g., Rogers, Singer, & Imperio, 1993), there seems little doubt that press attention helped to educate Americans about AIDS. As noted in the previous chapter, spectacular media coverage of Magic Johnson's disclosure helped to transform public perceptions of AIDS, bringing a sensitive issue into mainstream public discussion. Were it not for the media, people would not know about AIDS, its devastating effects on poor communities, and how to protect themselves from HIV infection.

However, there have been disturbing disparities between perceptions and knowledge, with certain groups more knowledgeable about AIDS than others. This is consistent with the **knowledge gap hypothesis,** which stipulates that the infusion of media information increases knowledge disparities between richer, more educated individuals and their poorer, less educated counterparts. As discussed in chapter 4, poor minority women frequently harbor misconceptions about HIV transmission, both because they do not have as much access to information about AIDS as other individuals, and because they perceive that AIDS messages featuring dissimilar others are not so relevant to their needs. It is likely that the knowledge gap between rich and poor people is even greater in Third World countries, where access to media is more stratified.

Another area in which media have had an impact is on attitudes toward individuals suffering from AIDS, particularly gay men who have contracted the disease. Stories about the plight of gay men with AIDS and the extensive care these individuals have received from their lovers have probably helped change attitudes toward homosexual men, perhaps by increasing empathy for gay men and redefining the gay identity in the public mind from one based exclusively on sex to one founded on a larger human identity (Herek, 1997).

Interpersonal Communication. Once knowledge has been acquired from mass media, people can begin to contemplate ways of combining knowledge with feelings and acting on what they have learned. According to diffusion theory, interpersonal communication is instrumental in persuading people to adopt an innovation. This is congenial with the approach taken in this book, which has emphasized the myriad ways in which individuals influence one another to adopt or resist safer sex change. Interpersonal communication in AIDS prevention campaigns frequently takes the form of street outreach activities, small-group discussions, classroom instruction, and peer counseling (Rogers & Shefner-Rogers, 1999).

Diffusion theory also stresses the role played by **homophily,** or similarity between communicator and message recipient (Dearing, Meyer, & Rogers, 1994). The more that the change agent can convey to message recipients that he or she shares their values, language, and ways of seeing the world, the more successful the leader is apt to be. As one staff member in a prevention program geared to gay Native Americans said, "I think this is pretty basic for us, the philosophy of Natives helping Natives, and we got 100% Native staff, 100% Native board, most of our volunteers are Native, and it's really about hearing the information coming from another Native gay man" (Dearing et al., 1996, p. 357). Making matters more complicated, there are also instances in which members of the community group disagree among themselves and cases in which community groups advocate positions that are incompatible with the goals of public health (see Bayer, 1994 and discussion that follows).

Social Marketing

While diffusion theory calls on communication principles, social marketing applies marketing ideas to devise prosocial programs. *Social marketing* is defined as **"a process of designing, implementing, and controlling programs to increase the acceptability of a prosocial idea among population segments of consumers"** (Dearing et al., 1996, p. 345). The creative aspect of social marketing is that it applies techniques developed to promote commercial products to an entirely different context: campaigns to promote prosocial causes. This is not a simple application because social and commercial marketing differ in important ways. Social marketers are not motivated by profit but by a desire to improve the lot of others, some of whom may not want to change their "lot" at all. In addition, social marketing efforts are frequently directed at the poorest and least educated members of society, who are more difficult to reach than the middle-class consumers targeted by commercial campaigns (Ratzan & Payne, 1993).

Social marketing is akin to, yet different from, persuasion. Like persuasion, it attempts to change people's minds, relying not on coercion but on the tools of communication and self-influence. Unlike interpersonal persuasion, social marketing attempts to achieve change by using macro resources: community organizations, political institutions, and mass media. In addition, social marketing is based on the assumption that you must provide people with a worthwhile product or service in exchange for their participation in the program. "Something of value must be transferred or traded between parties who each benefit," note June Flora and her colleagues (Flora, Schooler, & Pierson, 1997, p. 362).

In the area of AIDS prevention, social marketing campaigns are complicated by four factors. First, as Edward Maibach, Gary Kreps, and Ellen Bonaguro (1993) note, "because the individuals who are at greatest risk for HIV/AIDS contagion are diverse, both culturally and behaviorally, it is unlikely that campaign planners can develop a general set of effective campaign messages that will work equally well with all audiences" (p. 16).

Second, individuals most at risk are typically the hardest to reach with persuasive messages. This is a standard problem in social marketing campaigns, but is particularly relevant in the case of AIDS campaigns. Individuals are sometimes afraid to attend informational meetings because they fear they will be branded an "AIDS victim," a label that can lead to social ostracism in certain American and African communities (Daley, 1998). A poor minority woman may be afraid that her boyfriend will infer from her attending a meeting that she has AIDS or is sleeping around, consequences that could threaten the relationship.

Third, certain AIDS prevention communications are likely to be seen as inappropriate or in bad taste by the public, which has not always empathized with the plight of those who suffer from HIV/AIDS (Maibach et al., 1993, p. 17). Television stations have been reluctant to air hard-hitting ads about condom use or to depict characters in dramatic series using or talking about condoms. By contrast, the same TV stations air hundreds of commercials showing sexually explicit images (Reichert et al., 1999) and broadcast passionate lovemaking (Greenberg & Busselle, 1996), typically without onscreen breaks for condom discussions. The news media have long avoided explicit references to risky sexual practices like "anal intercourse" and "swallowing semen" (Netter, 1992).

Fourth, value and political disagreements complicate efforts to seamlessly execute AIDS marketing campaigns. Campaigns directed at injecting drug users, taking heed of the difficulty of stopping addicts from injecting drugs, have opted for the more modest goal of inducing them to use bleach to disinfect needles or to exchange HIV-infected needles for sterile ones. This way, even if people keep hurting themselves through drugs, they won't die of HIV infection. However, these programs have been fought by political groups who fear that needle exchange will increase drug use. Although studies show that needle exchange programs have not had this effect, political opposition to such programs complicates the development of marketing campaigns directed at injecting drug users (Donovan, 1999).

In a similar fashion, safer sex campaigns have raised the ire of critics on both the Right and Left. Conservative partisans, some of whom harbor antigay biases (Herek & Capitanio, 1999), cringe at the thought that safer sex PSAs could show gay men in explicitly sexual positions. By the same token, gay leaders initially rejected the idea that AIDS should be framed as a virus affecting gay men (Fumento, 1990). Fearing that the label would further stigmatize homosexuals, they urged that AIDS be viewed as a disease affecting the United States as a whole. Such feelings make sense, in view of the prejudice gay men have faced. However, the danger is that by minimizing the degree to which the epidemic affected men who have sex with other men, activists did their brothers a disservice (Rotello, 1997).

More recently, AIDS activists have diverged on the value of the popular red lapel ribbon. Some organizers promote the use of this visual symbol as a gentle way to remind people of the continued suffering of people with AIDS, or "as a way of introducing public discussion of AIDS into places from which it has been previously excluded" (Sobnosky & Hauser, 1999, p. 26). On the other hand, other activists argue that ribbons "offer an easy way out of the AIDS crisis, as people adopt red ribbons as fashion accessories, largely devoid of any connection to the AIDS crisis" (Sobnosky & Hauser, 1999, p. 33).

The foregoing discussion underscores the role values play in AIDS prevention campaigns. The decision to mount a safer sex campaign is itself a value judgment because moral conservatives believe that condom education interferes with parental prerogatives and laissez-faire humanists feel that you shouldn't go around telling other people what to do. A message trying to teach condom-use skills may also affirm psychological solutions, perhaps suggesting that community-level action is less important than individual-level change (Guttman, 1997; Salmon, 1992). The groups marketers work with, constraints organizations place on campaign planners, decisions to focus on certain risk groups rather than others (or on risk groups rather than risky behaviors) all illustrate the pervasive role values play in social marketing campaigns.

Social Marketing Campaign Principles

Maibach and his colleagues (1993) argue that there are five stages in health communication campaigns: planning, application of theory, communication analysis, implementation, and evaluation and reorientation (see Fig. 6.1).

During the first phase, **planning,** practitioners set realistic goals for changing AIDS prevention attitudes and behaviors. Setting goals is not easy. Many questions arise. Should the campaign try to encourage individuals to contemplate the possibility that they are susceptible to HIV, teach behavioral skills, or induce long-term behavioral change? What counts as a success? Is it realistic to expect inexpensive social marketing interventions to produce large or even modest effects (Fishbein, 1996; Salmon, 1992)? Do social scientific studies have the power to detect small, but socially important, effects? Goals should be selected carefully, on the basis of the audience a campaigner wants to reach and what can be reasonably attained, based on research.

The second stage involves use of **theory.** Theory helps practitioners devise strategies, modify appeals, and predict the impact a campaign will have on a target audience's attitudes and behavior. A variety of theories can be applied, including cognitive decision, social psychological, and interpersonal communication approaches discussed in this book. An alternative approach, popular with some, is postmodernism, a pastiche of points of view that questions the very notion that communication stimuli have a certain meaning that can be objectively analyzed. Postmodernism holds that there is no such thing as ultimate meaning and that meanings are endlessly constructed by message receivers, as a function of their values and those of the larger culture (e.g., Derrida, 1976; Sacks, 1996). According to postmodern approaches:

> What is true, correct, or valid (beautiful, appropriate, or desirable) depends on the context within which inquiry is situated. . . . In the postmodern world, value resides in consumption—one must experience the product before its gratification

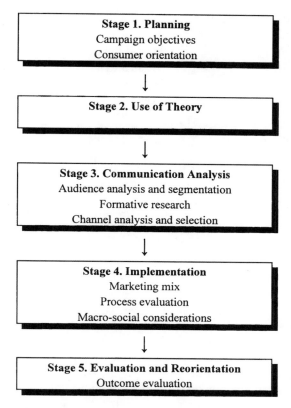

FIG. 6.1. A Strategic Health Communication Campaign Model. Adapted from "Developing strategic communication campaigns for HIV/AIDS prevention," (p. 19), by E. W. Maibach, G. L. Kreps, and E. W. Bonaguro. In S. Ratzan (Ed.), *AIDS: Effective Health Communication for the 90s,* 1993, Washington, DC: Taylor & Francis.

is apparent. The more consumers hold values that are contingent ("it all depends"), ideologically elusive ("don't ask me why; I don't know"), or diverse ("what's good for you may or may not be good for me"), the less they are likely to agree with broad public rationale; and, the less they are likely to accede to universal, societal prescriptions. (Kernan & Domzal, 1997, pp. 396–397, 399)

Postmodernism celebrates diversity—diversity of cultural groups and diversity of meanings assigned to communications. The implication for social marketing is that appeals viewed as didactic and moralistic will be rejected by postmodern consumers. So too will messages based on mainstream ideas and straightforward logic. Instead, ads that are "fast, giddy, clever, cynical, and full

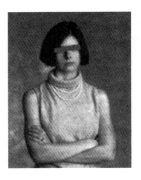

This is the girl,
Who's in love with a man,
Who picked someone up at a party,
Who'd been out with her boss,
Who'd taken a client to Hamburg,
Who'd suggested a tart,
Who'd been with an addict,
Who'd just shared a needle,
With a friend down the road,
Who had AIDS.

FIG. 6.2.   Postmodern ad on AIDS prevention. From "Hippocrates to Hermes: The postmodern turn in public health advertising" (p. 408), by J. B. Kernan and T. J. Domzal. In M. E. Goldberg, M. Fishbein, and S. E. Middlestadt (Eds.), *Social Marketing: Theoretical and Practical Perspectives,* 1997, Mahwah, NJ: Lawrence Erlbaum Associates.

of irony" will resonate with today's consumers (Kernan & Domzal, 1997, p. 400). Postmodernism is not a theory; it is full of ambiguities and contradictions that frustrate scholars who properly look for clarity and coherence. It shares features with cognitively oriented persuasion theories, but differs in key respects (not the least of which is that it frequently defies empirical testing).

Applied to AIDS campaigns, postmodernism suggests that social marketers should avoid preachy, "heavy-duty" fear appeals. They should recognize that the audience they are frequently trying to reach (disadvantaged, marginalized segments of society) are those who are especially sympathetic with a postmodern perspective. If audience members are to be persuaded, they must be engaged by ads that respect their individuality and irreverence for mainstream norms. Figure 6.2 illustrates a postmodern AIDS prevention ad.

Once they have applied theories to campaign development, practitioners move to the third phase of an AIDS prevention intervention: **communication analysis.** At this juncture, the emphasis is on analyzing the target audience and understanding its values. "Because a group's history, language, values, and beliefs influence group members' health-related knowledge, attitudes, and behavior," Flora and her colleagues (1997) note, "the values of a culture must be used as the foundation or building blocks of health promotion programs" (p. 356). Or as Ronald Bayer (1994) puts it, "AIDS prevention efforts that are not culturally sensitive will be ineffective" (p. 895).

During this third phase of a campaign, planners segment the audience into smaller, more homogeneous audience groups, capitalizing on the psychological principle of similarity or homophily. Formative research is conducted to understand audience members' HIV-related beliefs and their reactions to persuasive messages.

The campaign is launched during the fourth stage, **implementation**. Campaigns can involve PSAs, videos, brochures, and group sessions. The key element is the marketing mix—the four Ps of marketing: **product, price, placement,** and **promotion.** Let's go over each of these in turn.

Most of us do not associate *products* with prosocial campaigns. However, social marketing interventions promote numerous products. These can be material entities (condoms, bleach, red ribbons), slogans (Silence = Death), or ideas (advice on how to talk with a partner about safer sex).

Should marketers charge a *price* for condoms? Perhaps they should hand condoms out free, particularly to poor people. In some cases, this makes sense. In many contexts, however, social marketing organizations are advised to charge a price (Dahl, Gorn, & Weinberg, 1997). First, charging a price can help the organization cover costs of providing services. Second, price can motivate managers by offering them a financial incentive. Third, people tend to perceive products as having more value when there is cost associated with them.

Placement involves deciding where to place the AIDS prevention message. Which medium is best? Should a specialized medium be targeted? An Internet web site? If television is selected, what time of day is best to reach audience members? If the marketing organization can't afford television, what medium should it use instead? If research indicates that audience members have adequate knowledge and are in the persuasion stage of decision making, how should interpersonal communication be used to reach them? What types of opinion leaders would be most influential?

The Internet is becoming an increasingly important channel for AIDS campaign messages. It is especially useful in reaching those who have faced prejudice from mainstream society and feel more comfortable communicating in modalities that protect their privacy. In August 1999, six gay men who contracted syphilis reported that they had met their last sexual partners through an America Online (AOL) chat room, San Francisco Men 4 Men (Nieves, 1999b). In an effort to alert other chat room members of the health risk, AOL put the San Francisco public health department in touch with an online service for homosexuals, Planet Out. Planet Out in turn relied on e-mail and its web site to pass the word to chat room users, who would be especially likely to trust communications from the chat group.

Promotion is the final aspect of the marketing mix. It involves persuasion, all the theories discussed in this book, along with an appreciation of the different meanings audiences attribute to AIDS prevention. Think how differently condoms are perceived by social marketers, religious conservatives, sexually active young people, poor ethnic women, and people living in sex-positive subcultures. Language is important. Words carry symbolic meanings.

Case in point: Thirty years ago, campaign practitioners in India recognized that condoms had been known as "French letters" and were regarded as taboo. Social marketers renamed condoms Nirodh, from an Indian word meaning "protection." They test-marketed the product in New Delhi and successfully promoted it across the nation (Rogers, 1995). In Jamaica, the name Panther was chosen for condoms after marketing research suggested that the name had strong macho connotations (DeJong & Winsten, 1992). In Sri Lanka, Preethi ("beautiful") was selected. These names clearly have a lot more going for them than our home-grown American manufacturer's Trojan label!

It is important to remember that the four Ps of marketing do not take place in a vacuum. Social marketing campaigns are influenced by societal norms and a host of *macrosocial factors*. American society's hostility toward homosexuality has profoundly affected the dynamics of AIDS prevention campaigns directed at gay men. Media interventions targeted at gay men have little chance of getting aired on mainstream media, to say nothing of attracting funds from major funding organizations. In addition, our society's ambivalence about sexuality has hamstrung campaigners' ability to talk frankly with adolescents.

Complicating matters, different social groups view sex in profoundly different ways. The liberal culture embraces sex, but many working-class parents and religious groups believe that abstinence is preferable to safer sex, resent the intrusion of condom ads into their living rooms, and view condom education as infringing on parental prerogatives (Bayer, 1994). By contrast, in certain African countries safer sex campaigns are seen as threatening deep-seated beliefs in polygamy and promiscuity.

In addition to cultural mores and economic factors, subcultural values also influence campaigns directed at audience segments. For example, safer sex campaigns directed at gay men in San Francisco have been embroiled in subcultural controversy.

In the 1980s, many gay activists viewed bathhouses as one of the few places in society where they could be themselves, free of society's prejudices. Bathhouses were also sites of rampant promiscuity, with men practicing unsafe sex with as many as hundreds of different sexual partners, some of whom had contracted the AIDS virus (Rotello, 1997). While gay men viewed bathhouses in civil liberties terms, San Francisco health officials framed the issue in "communitarian" language (Etzioni, 1998), emphasizing the health of the larger community and dangers that unprotected bathhouse sex posed to the gay community and the city as a whole. After years of conflict between the city and bathhouse proponents, the two groups worked out a compromise. Sex clubs replaced bathhouses, and in the clubs sex is permitted so long as it is public and club monitors can assess whether partners are using condoms (Nieves, 1999a).

The compromise recently came under fire from gay activists who object to performing sex in front of other people and resent the attitude that gay men cannot be trusted to practice protected sex without being monitored. These individuals favor reopening the bathhouses, with the proviso that condoms and testing for STDs be widely available. However, public health proponents disagree. They argue that HIV prevention is more important than allowing gay people to express themselves sexually in every way. Both sides have a point. As one public health expert acknowledged, "this is a place where reasonable people who really do care about gay men's health can disagree in profound ways" (Nieves, 1999a, p. 9).

Social marketing campaigns directed at sexually active gay San Franciscans are caught between these two extremes. Efforts to accommodate community values are complicated when the community itself is divided and cultural sensitivity clashes with the larger goals of AIDS prevention (Bayer, 1994). In these cases, social marketers must be politicians as well as persuaders. They must find the region where they can be maximally effective and do the best they can, with specific, limited objectives. As Susan Middlestadt and her colleagues (1997) observe, marketers must "begin where the community is, get out of their way when assistance is not needed, and be available at the moment they do need it" (p. 310).

The final phase of a social marketing campaign is **evaluation and reorientation.** Practitioners must assess the impact of the campaign on targeted behaviors, look at positive, negative, intended, and unintended effects, decide what went right, what went wrong, and plan new AIDS prevention campaigns accordingly (see Dearing et al., 1998).

Summary. Social marketing and diffusion of innovations contain useful suggestions for health practitioners. Neither is a panacea. Social marketing is not a theory that contains testable hypotheses for communication campaign design. Such hypotheses are found in persuasion models. Diffusion of innovations offers a more compelling theoretical perspective; however, it is difficult to locate the empirical basis of some of the theory's many generalizations. These limits notwithstanding, there is little doubt that both diffusion and social marketing help us bridge the micro and macro areas of AIDS prevention persuasion and offer provocative ideas for designing large-scale communication campaigns.

National AIDS Prevention Campaigns

Influenced by macro perspectives such as social marketing, the U.S. government and CDC have developed several national AIDS awareness campaigns. Back in 1987 and 1988, the Surgeon General and the CDC teamed up to develop an *America Responds to AIDS* campaign. *America Responds to AIDS* consisted of a series of televised public service announcements in which an individual who knew a person with AIDS discussed the virus, tried to arouse fear to motivate behavioral change, and emphasized the need to take precautions against HIV infection. The PSAs closed by giving a toll-free telephone number for viewers to call for additional information (Winett, Altman, & King, 1990). Later that year, the Surgeon General sent a brochure, *Understanding AIDS,* to all U.S. households in an effort to increase knowledge of AIDS transmission and prevention. Subsequently, other PSAs targeted sexually active women.

The campaign was "precedent setting," noted Richard Winett and his colleagues (1990). It was the first time that television networks and cable stations conducted a prolonged health-information campaign on AIDS and safer sex. Theory and research suggest that *America Responds to AIDS* had several beneficial effects (Siska et al., 1992; Snyder, 1991). The campaign succeeded in:

1. Stimulating interest in AIDS prevention, as measured by calls to the National AIDS Hotline.
2. Strengthening perceptions that AIDS was a national problem.
3. Sparking discussions about AIDS among family members.

Unfortunately the campaign had liabilities, including the following:

1. There was little effort to segment the audience into major at-risk groups, with few specialized messages directed at gay men, injecting drug users, or poor women.
2. Few communications discussed condom use explicitly and persuasively.
3. There was little attention paid to modeling strategies to help people talk more comfortably about safer sex.
4. The campaign did not adequately link up with community organizations and neighborhood opinion leaders who might influence individuals at risk for HIV infection.

More than a decade later, barriers still exist in using the media to promote AIDS prevention (Romer & Hornik, 1992; Walters, Walters, & Priest, 1999). The cost of purchasing broadcast time exceeds the budget of most health education organizations, and television stations are still nervous about airing hard-hitting condom ads. The best bet is to take a more intensive focus and direct campaigns at specialized groups, using appropriate communication channels. As it turns out, a variety of targeted interventions have been developed, and some have been remarkably successful. In the next section, I discuss these campaigns in an effort to showcase ways that communication can be used to influence AIDS prevention behaviors, and to offer theory-based suggestions to improve communication campaigns. The discussion is organized around groups at risk to contract the AIDS virus.

RECEIVER FACTORS:
EFFECTS OF SPECIALIZED CAMPAIGNS

Heterosexual College Students and Teenagers

There is strong empirical evidence that interventions can change young people's HIV-related attitudes and behaviors. It can be done! Fisher and Fisher (1993, 1996) conducted a series of interventions, testing their Information–

Motivation–Behavioral Skills (IMB) Model on diverse student samples (see chapter 5). They typically assign one group of students the IMB experimental materials and earmark another group as the no-treatment control condition. The intervention consists of *information* (an "AIDS 101 Slide Show" that provides facts about HIV transmission, corrects stereotypes about partner risk, and offers information about AIDS prevention). The project targets *motivation* through a documentary, "People Like Us," that features interviews with six HIV-infected young people who are similar to university students in appearance and background. The intervention also teaches *behavioral skills* through a humorous videotape ("Sex, Condoms, and Videotape") that models safer sex communication skills, as well as through peer education, and actual instruction in putting on condoms correctly (using a wooden replica of a penis!).

Research indicates that the intervention reduces misperceptions, leads to more favorable attitudes toward performing HIV-prevention behaviors, and increases condom purchases (Fisher & Fisher, 1996; for evidence of other successful HIV interventions, see Rotheram-Borus et al., 1998; Rothman et al., 1999; Sanderson & Jemmott, 1996; Weisse, Turbiasz, & Whitney, 1995).

The IMB research program tells us that practitioners can enhance AIDS prevention motivation and behaviors. However, this does not mean they will always succeed. Persuasive communications do not always work; they run up against a host of social psychological barriers, particularly when trying to reach college students and teenagers, who assume they are invulnerable to life's misfortunes.

Complicating matters, young people are desensitized to AIDS prevention messages, having been bombarded by them since elementary school. Carefully constructed communications that may be persuasive in other health domains can be easily discounted. Youthful audience members frequently interpret messages differently than middle-aged campaign planners. Not surprisingly, for example, a University of California at Santa Barbara student orientation video showed a man having sex with a different woman every weekend. After several months of this promiscuous sex, the man died. But the message failed to arouse fear because, as one student put it, "you're not thinking, 'I'm scared of getting one of those diseases.' You're thinking, 'Wow if it's as easy as what they're saying, I want to get out there.' I mean the guy was just a regular-looking guy" (Lipsky, 1995, p. 82).

To motivate behavior change, fear appeals must do what the research says: target salient beliefs, arouse appropriate amounts of fear, and contain efficacy information (Struckman-Johnson & Struckman-Johnson, 1996; Witte, 1998). Messages must teach as well as scare. Campaigns geared to university students must be in sync with a freewheeling environment, in which students are sexually experienced, assume they're not personally at risk for STDs, combine sex with drinking, and discount HIV because it arouses defensiveness and they don't see much evidence of it around campus anyway. Postmodern PSAs that combine irreverence with compelling information can be particularly effective communication devices. Messages geared to adolescents can use humor to deflect tension, as in this radio spot:

> Remember how when you were a little kid your mom used to tell you, "Now, don't go out without your rubbers!" That's even better advice today. If you're going to have sex, play it safe. Use a latex condom with a spermicide containing Nonoxynol-9. For confidential help and information, call 1-800-872-AIDS. This message comes to you from the Michigan Department of Public Health AIDS Prevention Program. And your mom. (Romer & Hornik, 1992, p. 150)

The ad isn't perfect. Few listeners will remember the "Nonoxynol-9." Many will feel uncomfortable with the last line that connects their mothers with sexual intimacy. Nonetheless, the ad meshes with persuasion theory and succeeded in increasing awareness of an AIDS Hotline and enhancing key beliefs (Romer & Hornik, 1992).

One strategy that is apt to be particularly effective among high school and college students is to target perceived group norms (DiClemente, 1992b; Fisher, Misovich, & Fisher, 1992; Ratzan & Payne, 1993; Winslow, Franzini, & Hwang, 1992). Because it is difficult to shatter perceptions of invulnerability, practitioners might take a more indirect tack. They might point out that, contrary to popular belief, many young people actually endorse HIV prevention and would use condoms if a partner requested it. This would help break the mutual silence that occurs when each partner incorrectly assumes the other won't use condoms. In a similar fashion, peer educators could try to correct the inaccurate perception many men hold—that broaching the condom topic will reduce their sexual attractiveness. In fact, women view guys who have condoms available as behaving sensibly and responsibly, a perception that probably increases men's sexual appeal (Galligan & Terry, 1993).

In high schools, peer strategies can be particularly effective. Some educators argue that interventions geared at teenagers should do more than advocate safer sex and must recommend "truly 100% safe sex"; in other words, abstinence (Emenike, 1997, p. 325). Teens who are slightly older than the targeted group may be particularly credible speakers in campaigns trying to persuade students to postpone sexual intercourse.

Humor can also be effective. In a campaign geared to Seattle adolescents, Alstead and his colleagues (1999) carefully matched message appeals to perceived barriers to condom use. They also devised some funny communications. For example, a bus sign featured a child's picture and the words:

250,000 TIMES CHEAPER!!
. . . Than the Average Child!
CONDOMS
They Go Where You Go.

A billboard showed a macho-looking man holding a rubber. The caption read:

4 OUT OF 4
. . . People Surveyed PREFER
Condoms Over Herpes!!!

The campaign succeeded in reaching a high percentage of target adolescents and stimulated discussion.

Summary. Adolescents and college students continue to be an important audience for HIV preventive messages. The teen years in particular are a time of great sexual experimentation. What's more, adolescents perceive they are invulnerable to health risks, large numbers of teenagers across economic classes practice unprotected sex, and many teens believe that condoms reduce sexual pleasure or are embarrassing to obtain (Trad, 1994). These attitudes are particularly prevalent among runaway and homeless youths, a group at particular risk for HIV infection due to high-risk sexual practices, injection drug use, and lack of access to quality health care (Sondheimer, 1992). Social marketing strategies must continue to target teenagers, matching theory and strategy to a skeptical, but ultimately reachable, audience.

Gay Men

There is good news and bad news when it comes to campaigns directed at gay and bisexual men. The good news is that, beginning with the aggressive efforts of the San Francisco gay community in the 1980s, social interventions have profoundly changed gay men's sexual habits. The bad news is that, with many young gay men continuing to practice unsafe sex (see chapter 3), campaigns face daunting challenges if they are to maintain positive changes that have occurred.

During the 1980s, in the wake of epidemic-level increases in HIV infection among gay men, educators mounted multifaceted campaigns to raise awareness about AIDS and to teach men safer sex skills. The interventions, particularly those in San Francisco, succeeded in reducing incidence of high-risk sexual behaviors and in building social support for HIV prevention (Coates, 1990; Ekstrand & Coates, 1990). Efforts to influence risky behaviors made use of skills approaches (discussed in chapter 5), diffusion theory, and social marketing. Some of the earliest and most innovative studies of campaigns directed at gay men were conducted by Jeffrey Kelly and his colleagues.

In a micro-level study that applied behavioral skills principles, Kelly and his associates (1989) recruited 104 gay men with a history of risky sexual behavior to participate in an experimental intervention or to serve as control group subjects. The intervention consisted of 12 weekly group sessions led by two clinical psychologists. Experimental group participants discussed situations in which they had engaged in risky sexual activities, were taught to generate statements that emphasized performance of safer sex ("I will feel much better tomorrow if I don't do anything risky tonight"), were given instruction in how to turn down a partner's unsafe sex request, and role-played assertive safer sex responses.

The intervention increased knowledge about AIDS risks, enhanced safer sex assertiveness skills, and promoted use of safer sex alternatives. As Fig. 6.3 shows, experimental subjects also reduced their frequency of unprotected anal intercourse and increased condom use, relative to controls. For example, prior to the study both experimental and control group subjects used condoms 24% of all times when they had anal intercourse. Four months later, control group participants reported using condoms 19% of the time, whereas experimental group subjects increased condom use to 66% of all anal intercourse occasions. Condom use rose to 77% at an 8-month follow-up.

In a subsequent study, Kelly et al. (1991) applied diffusion theory principles to HIV risk reduction. Observing that opinion leaders (i.e., significant others) influence the adoption of innovations, the researchers recruited popular leaders among gay men in a small Mississippi city to help spread the word about HIV risk prevention.

Kelly and his associates identified leaders by asking bartenders at gay clubs to observe the men who were greeted most positively by patrons. Once leaders were identified, they were asked to participate in the intervention program. The opinion leaders subsequently discussed and modeled safer sex skills in conversations with patrons at the clubs. To stimulate conversation, posters with traffic light circles were placed in the clubs and leaders wore a lapel button with the same logo (red for high risk, yellow for moderate risk, and green for low risk). This invited questions and sparked discussion.

To examine effects of the intervention, researchers compared survey responses from gay club patrons in the experimental community (Biloxi, Mississippi) with those of men entering clubs in comparison communities (Hattiesburg, Mississippi and Monroe, Louisiana). The fact that men reported peer norms and sexual behavior anonymously in gay clubs gave the study a realistic edge.

The intervention succeeded in reducing the incidence of high-risk sex over a 2-month period. Roughly 9% fewer men engaged in anal intercourse in Biloxi, compared with 3% fewer in the comparison communities. Condom use in anal intercourse increased by 6.5% in Biloxi and declined by 6.1% in the two control cities.

To be sure, it's not known whether these changes persisted over time. Men in the intervention community may also have felt some pressure to report that they were engaging in safer sex, perhaps to please opinion leaders and researchers. Nonetheless, the findings are encouraging, suggesting that communication campaigns can change deep-seated sexual attitudes and behaviors if they are designed properly and take into account what practitioners know

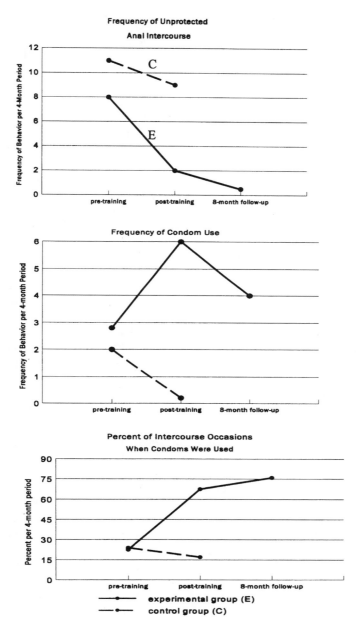

FIG. 6.3. Effects of an experimental intervention on protected and unprotected sex among gay men. From "Behavioral intervention to reduce AIDS risk activities," by J. A. Kelly, J. S. St. Lawrence, H. V. Hood, and T. L. Brasfield, 1989, *Journal of Consulting and Clinical Psychology, 57*, p. 65.

about the diffusion of innovations. Indeed, Kelly and his colleagues (1997) repli-
cated their 1991 findings in gay bars in eight communities across four regions of
the United States, using an even stronger experimental methodology.

A flurry of other macro-level studies, conducted with community-level support, also found that campaigns can reduce gay men's practice of risky sex (e.g.,
Kegeles, Hays, & Coates, 1996). Some might conclude from this, and the fading
of AIDS as a perceived national problem, that the battle against risky sex among
gay men has been fought and won. However, unsafe sexual practices continue
apace, particularly in smaller cities outside the AIDS epicenters (Coates, 1990;
Nieves, 1999a). Thus, it remains important to target gay and bisexual men with
persuasive interventions, guided by theory and implemented with up-to-date
social marketing techniques.

For those young men who seek pleasure and deny that they are at risk, campaigns should try to help them label their behavior as problematic and assist
them in contemplating changing high-risk behaviors. Fishbein and his colleagues
(1992) have argued that persuasion campaigns directed at gay men should take
into account the cohesiveness of the gay community. Fishbein and his associates
found that men living in a city with a well-organized gay community were more
influenced by social norms than those living in a city where the gay community
is primarily underground. In communities that can offer interpersonal support
for gay men, safer sex campaigns should highlight subjective norms, or the
opinions of influential others. In cities where the gay community is not so well
organized, campaigns should focus on attitudes, such as eroticizing safe sex,
while trying to gradually build a sense of community among gay men.

Practitioners must be careful not to legislate safer sex norms in a politically
correct manner. Instead, communications should emphasize that there is social
support for maintaining safer sex behaviors; at the same time, they should
respect individuals' struggles to engage in safer sex (Díaz, 1998). Campaign professionals must also recognize that the gay community is not a singular, homogeneous entity but a complex constellation with diverse subsets, such as gay
teenagers, older White and younger African American gay men, as well as bisexual men who would prefer their identity be closeted (Kelly, 1995). Because
each of these groups has different norms and perceptions of risk, campaigns
must employ different strategies to reach different subsets, utilizing social marketing segmentation principles. For example, interventions geared to bisexual
men must employ different strategies than those designed for openly gay men.
Bisexual men have lower condom use intentions and engage in riskier sex than
exclusively gay men (Heckman et al., 1995). Campaigns directed at bisexual
men are urgently needed because some bisexual men infected with HIV transmit the virus to women (Altman, 1999a).

Peer and community interventions are particularly important today, when
some gay men have developed an illusory belief that new drug therapies will
prevent the onset of HIV infection, thereby allowing them to engage in promis-

cuous unprotected sex. Drugs like protease inhibitors can help reduce the ravages of AIDS, but they are not panaceas and do not work equally well for all men under all circumstances (Altman, 1999a; Sternberg, 1999b).

Another problem is that sex is not always a rational act. Some gay men take sexual chances not because they lack knowledge of the risks but because unsafe sex satisfies important psychological needs, like companionship or escape from both tension aroused by AIDS and prejudices of mainstream U.S. society. Communications must convince men that they can satisfy their emotional longings in ways that do not put them in jeopardy of contracting the AIDS virus. Campaigns should use novel messages, in light of the "been there, done that" feeling that many gay men have toward condom messages that have been circulating in gay circles for nearly 20 years (Curtius, 1999).

The provision of social support can go a long way toward helping men develop the psychological fortitude that is needed to "say no" to the temptations of unsafe sex and to affirm a safe gay lifestyle (Seibt et al., 1995). Such support is especially important in Latino gay communities, where men need to overcome perceptions of low sexual control, as well as double binds created by parents who love their sons deeply but believe that homosexuality is sinful (Díaz, 1997). Communication campaigns are important here, but are not the entire answer. Communication and marketing work alongside and within a nexus of macrosocial forces, and the latter must be influenced if genuine social change is to occur. Rotello (1997) has persuasively argued that the gay community must create a new social structure that rewards self-restraint, long-term relationships, and "the whole human being" rather than sexual adventurism and risk-taking. He points out that:

> Logic would . . . suggest that if gay men want to create a sustainable culture, [the] reward system has to be turned upside down. Taking a lesson from environmentalism and population control, immediate and tangible social rewards need to be implemented to encourage safety and restraint. And these rewards will have to be built right into the structure of gay society if they are to effectively counterbalance the weak penalties and strong rewards that currently help to foster a culture of risk among many gay men. . . . If the central task of the new gay male culture is the integration of sexuality into a whole life, a life that respects sex but does not make it the central point of existence, gay culture needs to embrace the whole human being, his spiritual and personal self, his humanity, his vocations, his dreams, and not just his muscles or his libido or his penis. It has to draw explicit connections between sex and intimacy, and needs to reward self-restraint and end the pervasive belief that those who are living at the most extreme fringes of gay sexual life are somehow the most liberated and the most gay. (p. 244)

Toward this end, Rotello argues that gay communities devise alternatives to bars as the major place for gay men to meet. He also advocates gay marriage, noting that the marriage contract contains a powerful expectation that partners will remain faithful to one another. Although gay marriage, like heterosexual marital union, does not prevent sexual infidelity, it offers rewards for remaining faithful and provides disincentives for unsafe sex outside the relationship. What's more, if society allowed gay men to raise children, they could experience joys that would replace the sense of excitement unsafe sex offers; the selflessness required to raise children could take the place of the unbridled selfishness that gives rise to endless promiscuous sex.

It is noteworthy that this argument was made by a writer (Rotello) who has long been a gay activist and is familiar with the excessive sexual experimentation that occurred in the 1970s and 1980s. When a gay partisan argues that it is time to put a rein on sexual promiscuity and makes a case for a conservative institution—marriage—it seems to me that the argument is especially compelling and worthy of consideration.

Ethnic Minorities

"Effective persuasive campaigns require an insider's familiarity with the values and attitudes of the target audience," observes Patrick McLaurin (1995, p. 302). "In addition," McLaurin notes, "campaigns that attempt to influence by modeling the new behaviors must be aware of the norms of social interaction particular to the culture." His comments apply to AIDS prevention campaigns in general, but are particularly relevant to those directed at African Americans and ethnic minorities. Individuals from these groups have distinctive ways of interpreting persuasive messages based on their values and cultural history.

Campaigns that have recognized the need to tailor programs to cultural demands have succeeded in modifying AIDS-related behaviors (Jemmott, 1996; Myrick, 1998; NIMH, 1998; Peterson, 1997). For example, John Jemmott and his colleagues (1992) developed a series of interventions geared to inner-city Black adolescents that make use of culturally appropriate media materials. He shows teens a video, *The Subject is AIDS,* that is narrated by an African American woman and features a multiethnic cast. He engages them in a game, "AIDS Basketball," that gives kids points for correctly answering questions about AIDS prevention. Jemmott reports that his interventions have lowered intentions to engage in risky sexual behaviors and resulted in increases in safer sexual practices.

McLaurin (1995) argues that campaigns directed at inner-city African Americans must take several unique aspects of the culture into account. These include Black culture's oral tradition, which emphasizes metaphor, storytelling, and dynamic interaction between speaker and listener; its oppositional nature (objection to mainstream society's values); and fascination with hip-hop music. Campaigns must do more than call on same-race role models. Role models who appealed to these young people's parents would have little effect on the kids themselves, some of whom are so alienated from mainstream politics that they were unable to tell McLaurin the names of the African American mayors of their cities. Rather than relying on older Black celebrities, campaign planners should select communicators who are viewed as credible by the youthful target audience. Musicians like Puff Daddy or Public Enemy's Chuck D or Foxy Brown would resonate with a younger inner-city Black audience.

As a general rule, media role models and movies seen as coming from inside the culture will influence minority youth's attitudes toward AIDS prevention. McLaurin found that many of the teenagers he interviewed learned that HIV could be spread through oral sex from an incidental conversation between a main character and his "posse" in the movie *Boyz-N-the-Hood*. "We found it hard to believe, given the money that has been spent on HIV information campaigns, that this could be considered new information," McLaurin notes, adding that "when pressed, however, the teens admitted that although they had heard this before, the movie really made them believe it" (p. 318). In persuasion theory terms, the information was not persuasive and retrievable from memory unless delivered by a source in a context that was believable and perceived as authentic by the message receivers.

In his paper on persuasion and African American at-risk youths, McLaurin offers several recommendations for designing health communications. The suggestions, which are highly relevant for AIDS prevention campaigns, include the following:

1. Separate rejection of antisocial behavior from rejection of culture.
2. When and if possible, use street-accepted icons modeling desired behaviors and attitudes.
3. Messages must be directed at specific target audiences, not Black youths in general.
4. Media channels should not be perceived as being co-opted by the mainstream.
5. Media channels must have ability to be as current as tomorrow's fads. (p. 321)

Low-Income Women

There are many reasons why poor ethnic women choose unsafe sex. As discussed in chapter 4, poverty and drug abuse lead women to minimize risks of HIV infection. Economic inequality leaves women dependent on men for economic opportunities, which can put them at the mercy of sexually abusive men. Condoms can threaten a heterosexual relationship by bringing to mind fears that partners are cheating on one another. Since so many of these barriers to AIDS risk reduction are rooted in culture and systemic factors, one should not expect psychological interventions to work miracles. Nonetheless, individual-level and community-based interventions can effect change, and several treatments have helped to reduce sexual risk-taking.

John Jemmott, Loretta Jemmott, and their colleagues (1992) found that a series of games, role-playing, and educational exercises (one involving placing a condom on a banana!) led to increases in condom-use intentions. Jeffrey Kelly and his associates (1994) reported that safer sex skills training enhanced women's sexual communication skills, leading to significant increases in the use of condoms during vaginal intercourse.

Community-level campaigns have also been developed to influence low-income women. Kathleen Sikkema and Jeffrey Kelly (1995) took a social marketing approach, using outreach workers, social networking, and community activities such as educational parties and picnics, as well as communication skills training, to influence women living in low-income housing developments. The intervention enhanced AIDS prevention knowledge, sparked AIDS discussions, and significantly increased condom use (see Kalichman, 1998).

Unfortunately, interventions such as these are the exception, not the rule, in low-income communities. There are several reasons for this, including difficulty of obtaining funding for campaigns directed at low-income women, reluctance of mass media executives to develop communications directed at this audience segment, community resistance, and women's own fear of changing their personal lives. However, there is one bright spot on the horizon.

Recently, a female condom has been introduced. Sometimes termed a "vaginal pouch," **the female condom** "is a soft lubricated loose-fitting polyurethane pouch that lines the vagina" and has a soft ring at each end, with the closed ring used for insertion into the vagina. A new condom must be inserted each time a woman has sex (El-Bassel et al., 1998, p. 465). Although approved by the U.S. Food and Drug Administration in 1993, the device has been slow to gain in acceptability, and many people are unaware that it exists. Yet when compared to the male condom, the female condom has several advantages, including greater control by women, less risk of breakage, and coverage of the urethra which provides entrance for infections. In addition, because it does not require an erect penis for use, the device can reduce sexual anxiety, which occurs with the male condom when guys worry that they will lose their erection and women fret that if this occurs, guys will not like them.

Like all innovations, the female condom faces resistance. As one inner-city health clinic patient told researchers, "it looks like a garbage bag" (El-Bassel et al., p. 470). After discussing the condom in a focus group and subsequently using it during sex, respondents in Nabila El-Bassel and her colleagues' study changed their attitudes. One woman's comment was typical. "I loved the female condom, because you feel everything during sex," she said. "My partner loved it too because he had more space. It is not like the male condom which can be limiting to a man" (El-Bassel et al., p. 472). Male participants also reported that sex was more "fun" with the female condom.

The device is not without drawbacks. Some women told El-Bassel and her colleagues that they were uncomfortable inserting a strange object into their body or touching their genitals. Men interviewed in another study complained that the female condom was hard to use, or lamented that it put sexual power in the women's hands when "the man should be using the condom and not the woman" (Seal & Ehrhardt, 1999, p. 102). This may be a particularly common objection among men involved in relationships with women who use crack-cocaine (Ashery et al., 1995). Nonetheless, the greater control that the female condom affords women is a major plus, particularly for women who shy away from asking men to use a condom.

What's more, the new device has potential to increase AIDS preventive behavior in developing countries. The female condom is catching on in South Africa, a country ravaged by AIDS (McNeil, 1999). AIDS prevention workers are approaching prostitutes in Cape Town and handing out presents—free female condoms. "I've been using it since Valentine's Day, and I like it," a prostitute told a *New York Times* reporter (McNeil, 1999, p. A6). "It's quite great." The sex worker, whose husband is out of work and who has six children, adds that when men refuse to put on a condom, she goes into a bathroom and inserts the vaginal pouch. "They never know," she says. Her views were echoed by AIDS specialists working in Africa, who say they are astounded by its popularity.

Theories discussed in this book can help practitioners devise campaigns to promote the female condom. The Health Belief Model suggests that interventions emphasize the ways in which the female condom overcomes perceived barriers to safer sex. Social cognitive theory emphasizes that communicators should help people increase their self-efficacy or perception that they are capable of regularly using the vaginal pouch. Diffusion theory suggests that campaigns stress the degree to which the female condom offers people valuable benefits, is easy to use, and allows people to enjoy protected sex. Campaigns can also be useful in clearing up misconceptions, for example, the female condom does not work, it should be used with a male condom, or it is too small for a man's penis (Seal & Ehrhardt, 1999).

In the final analysis, interventions geared to women, particularly low-income minority women, will succeed to the degree that they take into account how women view safer sex. As functional theory reminds us, practitioners must appreciate the many reasons why women choose unsafe sex and gear messages accordingly. Perhaps, as Sobo (1995) suggests, "condoms could be represented as symbolic of the true and loving relationships that many women strive for rather than as necessary armor to protect against partners who will surely cheat" (p. 185). Campaigns that adopt this approach will not work miracles; communications cannot, after all, end poverty nor change power relationships between men and women. They can teach and motivate people to change sexual attitudes, and given the increasing numbers of infections among women in the United States, these are important objectives.

Injecting Drug Users and Sex Partners

A variety of interventions have been mounted to reach drug users and their sexual partners, two groups that are at risk for HIV infection and contain disproportionately high numbers of minority group members. According to researcher Richard Needle and colleagues (1998), these campaigns communicate the following message to IDUs: *"First, stop using and injecting drugs; if you cannot stop, use your own injection equipment and do not share it; if you must reuse or share injection equipment, disinfect with bleach to reduce transmission of HIV"* (italics added, p. 7).

Campaign planners have called on diffusion theory concepts as well as source credibility research. Practitioners take pains to hire outreach workers who live in the community at risk, who frequently talk with drug users and share their attitudes (Guenther-Grey et al., 1996). Former drug users can be particularly credible with IDUs because they speak the same language and offer first-hand evidence that it is possible to give up drugs. Psychologically oriented approaches suggest that campaigns match persuasive appeals to the individual's stage of change. For drug users who are contemplating a change in behavior, such as disinfecting needles with bleach, emotional messages may be most effective. For those who have already changed and are trying to maintain consistency, action-oriented communications may be more helpful (Fishbein & Guinan, 1996; Fishbein et al., 1997).

Some years back, I helped devise a campaign to influence inner-city drug users and their sexual partners (Perloff, 1991; Perloff & Pettey, 1991). We drew on fear communication theories to develop campaign strategies and called the campaign Project SAFE (Stay AIDS Free through Education). A brochure geared to drug users explained the risks that AIDS posed and provided a step-by-step diagram of how bleach could be used to clean dirty needles. A brochure directed at sex partners stressed that sexual partners were at risk for getting AIDS and offered explicit instructions on how to use a condom. Black-and-white posters with a picture of a tombstone and the inscription, "Don't Share a Bed with Someone Who Shares a Needle," were placed on buses, the rapid transit, and on billboards in inner-city neighborhoods. Interpersonal communication techniques supplemented the media campaign. A well-marked van distributed brochures, condoms, and a comic book that graphically described the risks AIDS posed to drug users (see Figs. 6.4 and 6.5). All materials prominently displayed the Project SAFE name and a hotline number.

The campaign increased awareness of Project SAFE and enhanced the belief that AIDS was a serious problem. Although it did not significantly increase knowledge of AIDS prevention, the campaign stimulated calls to the Project SAFE hotline.

In low-income urban areas, female sex partners of injecting drug users continue to be at risk for HIV infection. Even taking into account all of what is known about campaigns, it remains difficult to reach these women. They are

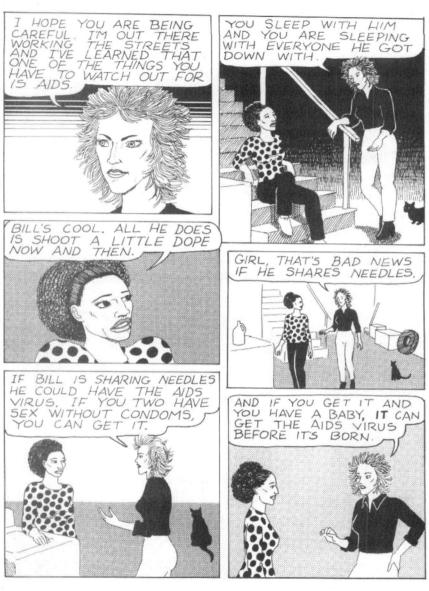

FIG. 6.4.   AIDS prevention comic strip geared to sex partners of injecting drug users. Reprinted from The Works: Drugs, Sex & AIDS, San Francisco AIDS Foundation.

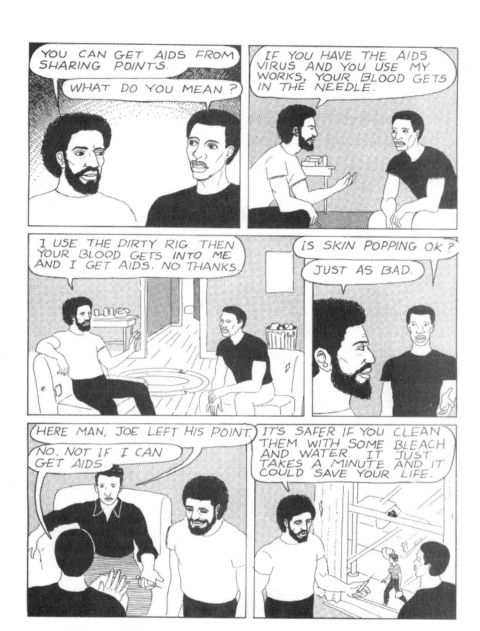

FIG. 6.5.   AIDS prevention comic strip directed at injecting drug users. Reprinted from The Works: Drugs, Sex & AIDS, San Francisco AIDS Foundation.

frequently hidden and hard to access through sex partners, community networks, or mass media (Krauss et al., 1999). Even when communications do modify attitudes, it remains difficult to ensure that short-term changes will last over a longer time. Unfortunately, female sex partners remain, as Lamptey and Weir (1992) put it, a "submerged part of the iceberg" (p. 170).

International Campaigns

HIV is spreading at literally epidemic proportions through Southeast Asia. There are 6.7 million HIV/AIDS cases in South and Southeast Asia, and the number is expected to grow (Altman, 1998). Thailand has been particularly hard hit, due to the large number of drug addicts, a hugely popular commercial sex industry, and a sexually active gay population. AIDS has been detected in every region of Thailand. In this country of 62 million, more than 800,000 persons are infected with the virus, approximately 1.25% of the populace (Svenkerud & Singhal, 1998). During the late 1980s and early 1990s, HIV spread among injecting drug users and also from female commercial sex workers to their male clients, who transmitted it to wives and sex partners. Thailand is also one of the few countries to have launched a series of government-run AIDS prevention campaigns, beginning in 1987 and continuing to the present (Pisalsarakit & Tillinghast, 1999). The Thai interventions are among the best documented in the world and offer a useful case study of social marketing of AIDS prevention (Steinfatt & Mielke, 1999).

Recognizing that the country faced an AIDS epidemic, the government launched a massive public health campaign in 1989. Sixty million condoms were distributed to more than 6,000 commercial sex establishments. Campaign planners encouraged brothel owners to require that sex workers engage only in protected sexual intercourse. The most popular prostitutes, called "superstars," received training in condom use and taught other workers these techniques. Condom use in sex establishments increased from approximately 6% to as much as 90% in some provinces (Steinfatt & Mielke, 1999). The number of STD cases dropped dramatically in the early 1990s.

The government simultaneously launched a media campaign geared to the general public. This featured short television spots, minidramas, documentaries, and billboards. Unfortunately, some messages indirectly blamed at-risk groups, such as commercial sex workers and drug users. Practitioners also neglected interpersonal communications, failing to call on grass roots agencies and sexual skills counseling.

In response to these deficiencies and growing numbers of HIV infections, campaign planners have modified their approach. They are supplementing mass media messages with interpersonal communication. They are working actively with secondary schools, factories, and community agencies, as diffusion and social marketing theories suggest. A "Wednesday Friends" club for HIV-infected people features healthy-looking speakers who disclose that they are HIV-positive during the course of their presentations. The revelation has a tremendous effect on listeners (Pisalsarakit & Tillinghast, 1999), mirroring the effects that a healthy-looking Magic Johnson had on American audiences and promoting identification between communicators and message receivers.

In poor Bangkok communities, a network of volunteers and peer opinion leaders offer AIDS prevention information to community members. Meetings take place on a soccer field. Instructional techniques run the gamut from traditional lecture-discussion to less conventional strategies, like a condom blowing competition for children. In other regions, practitioners have been nothing if not creative, setting up condom relay races in which relay teams put condoms on wooden penis models while blindfolded (Elkins et al., 1998)!

As Pim Pisalsarakit and Diana Tillinghast point out, these campaigns have had significant effects. Media publicity led to massive increases in knowledge about AIDS prevention. Some interventions enhanced condom use self-efficacy, whereas others have produced significant increases in condom use in sex establishments. More generally, Thai men are reassessing their free-wheeling attitudes toward sex and women's roles. Women are becoming increasingly aware of the threat AIDS poses to them and are organizing themselves to gain a greater sense of psychological empowerment.

Unfortunately, problems remain. HIV infection rates have not dropped as much as health educators would like. Double standards for male and female sexuality persist. The commercial sex industry continues to prosper, as it serves important functions for women and a Thai society that continues to treat women as sexual commodities (Chay-Nemeth, 1998). Even so, the Thai campaigns have shown an impressive ability to change in the face of negative feedback and, imperfect as they are, they remain as models for HIV-ravaged Southeast Asia.

The African situation, discussed in chapter 4, is a different story. As the number of HIV infections soars, the situation grows bleaker by the day. Campaigns have been launched in Africa, with some degree of success. However, campaign planners have failed to appreciate the perspectives of those at risk for HIV, and have been frustrated by lack of support from key decision makers (Lamptey & Weir, 1992). The only hope is for governments to take an active role in AIDS prevention interventions and to devote considerable community resources to the task. Although discussion of this issue is beyond the scope of this book, it bears repeating that campaigns must be based on theory, nurtured by intuitive community-honed appreciation for how target audience members think about the problem, and strengthened by coordination among government, community organizations, and people at risk for AIDS.

CONCLUSION

This chapter has reviewed AIDS prevention campaigns. I have discussed ways in which communication channels can be used to communicate HIV prevention information and explored strategies to reach diverse audience groups. Two macro-level theories have guided campaigns: diffusion theory and social marketing.

Diffusion theory examines the role communication plays in the spread of innovations. In the United States the media have had complex effects on AIDS prevention. The media helped to educate Americans about AIDS. At the same time, information has not diffused equally to all social groups, and the media have been reluctant to broadcast hard-hitting, but much needed, information about unsafe sex. Interpersonal communication plays an important role in the persuasion stage of AIDS prevention decision making. Diffusion theory calls attention to the ways in which homophily and opinion leadership influence people's decision making about safer sex issues.

Social marketing is a process of devising and implementing programs to increase acceptance of prosocial ideas. It emphasizes the role played by the four Ps of marketing—product, price, placement, and promotion—in the selling of AIDS prevention ideas and techniques. The four Ps do not take place in a vacuum. Social marketing campaigns are powerfully influenced by societal norms and a host of macrosocial factors. These factors include the nature of the economic system, media structure, cultural norms regarding sex, and community prejudices and predilections.

There are five stages in AIDS prevention campaigns: planning, theory application, communication analysis, implementation, and evaluation. Practitioners emphasize that communication campaigns must work closely with community groups, a task that is complicated when grass roots organizations disagree and advocate goals that pose a danger to the public health.

Over the past decades, there have been numerous AIDS prevention interventions at national, local and community levels. The first national campaign in the United States, *America Responds to AIDS,* stimulated interest in AIDS prevention. Yet planners failed to direct different messages to diverse at-risk segments and did not work adequately with community groups. In recent years, campaigns in the United States and abroad have targeted a variety of at-risk groups, such as sexually promiscuous heterosexual young people, gay men, injecting drug users and poor ethnic women. Interventions succeeded to the degree that they have called on social psychological and communication theories, and have linked up with grass roots organizations.

As HIV continues to infect people, particularly in the Third World where the disease is destroying economies and wiping out populations, information campaigns will become increasingly necessary. If they are to succeed, these campaigns must draw on persuasion theory and intelligently link up psychological concepts with larger community issues.

CHAPTER SEVEN

AIDS Stigma and Persuasion

> *If we assume that, as with cancer, most treatments will prolong life rather than cure the disease; if we assume that scientific research will continue to expand our knowledge rather than soon provide a means of prevention or cure; and if we assume that we will continue to respond to AIDS through the provision of specialized hospital units, long-term care, and other institutional services, we must also conclude that we are dealing not with a brief, time-limited epidemic but with a long, slow process more analogous to cancer than to cholera.* (Fee & Fox, 1992, p. 5)

HIV/AIDS will be with us for a while. People will contract HIV and gradually learn to integrate the virus into their everyday lives, surviving as best they can through a combination of drug therapy and old-fashioned optimism. The fortunate ones will live productive lives; the less fortunate will die soon after they contract the virus. This is another dimension of the AIDS pandemic, one with salient communication dimensions.

As it becomes increasingly common to know someone (or of someone) who has contracted HIV or AIDS, it becomes ever more important to teach people that AIDS is not a stigma or disfiguring mark, but rather a disease that calls for compassion and understanding.

This chapter focuses on the problem of AIDS stigma. Unlike previous chapters, this discussion does not focus on why people choose unsafe sex. In a sense, it does not concentrate so much on people who are at high risk for HIV infection, who may not be reading this book. Instead, it looks at us—the educated students and professionals who sometimes are not as fair-minded as we like to think we are. The chapter focuses on attitudes toward persons with AIDS (PWAs) and persons with HIV (PWHIVs). It examines why there is antipathy toward these individuals and suggests ways we can use persuasion to change public attitudes.

Note that I use the conventional term, persons with AIDS, rather than AIDS victims. People who contract HIV and get full-blown AIDS are in some sense victims, in the same way that someone who gets cancer or tuberculosis is a victim of an unfortunate life event. In addition, those who have AIDS are frequently victimized by society's prejudice. However, the term *victim* conveys that the individual is passive and helpless, which runs counter to what we know about those who have AIDS. It also suggests that these individuals are hapless and unable to run their lives, which is demonstrably false. For this reason, I rely on PWA terminology.

SOCIAL PSYCHOLOGY OF AIDS STIGMA

There is stigma associated with AIDS. You know what I mean if you feel uncomfortable thinking about the subject or shy away from articles in the media that deal with people with AIDS. You know what I mean if you would never shake the hand of someone who is infected with HIV, even though you rationally know you could not get the disease from a handshake.

In an ideal world, no one would look down on people with AIDS or view them as deviants to be avoided. Folks would empathize with PWAs, respecting their indomitable efforts to live their lives in the face of great stress. They would recognize that it is as ludicrous to think that someone with AIDS is morally bad as it is to believe that someone with polio or cancer or even syphilis is bad or flawed or inferior. But that is not what has happened. Too many of us, if we are honest with ourselves, harbor negative attitudes toward individuals who have contracted HIV/AIDS. Social psychologists would say we display AIDS stigma.

What is meant by *stigma?* The term originated with the Greeks, who viewed it as "a tattoo mark branded on the skin of an individual as a result of some incriminating action" (Crawford, 1996, p. 399). Nowadays, the term has a strong psychological dimension. Jones and his colleagues (1984) define the stigmatized as "the bearer of a 'mark' that defines him or her as deviant, flawed, limited, spoiled, or generally undesirable" (p. 6). Of course, there is nothing objectively wrong with the person; it is other people who supply the label and attach a negative meaning to whatever characteristic the individual possesses.

Unfortunately, AIDS is particularly likely to evoke stigma. As Gregory Herek (1999) explains:

> First, stigma is more often attached to a disease whose cause is perceived to be the bearer's responsibility. . . . Thus, because the primary transmission routes for HIV are behaviors that are widely considered voluntary and immoral, PWHIVs are regarded by a significant portion of the public as responsible for their condition and consequently are stigmatized. . . . Second, greater stigma is associated with illnesses and conditions that are unalterable or regenerative. Third, greater stigma is associated with conditions that are perceived to be contagious or to place others in harm's way. . . . Fourth, a condition tends to be more stigmatized when it is readily apparent to others—when it actually disrupts a social interaction or is perceived by others as repellent, ugly, or upsetting. . . . Given these characteristics, AIDS probably would have evoked stigma regardless of its specific epidemiology

and social history. Yet the character of AIDS stigma in the United States derives from the widely perceived association between HIV and particular sectors of the population, especially gay and bisexual men and injecting drug users (IDUs). (pp. 1109–1110)

Over the past decades, people with AIDS have been mocked, feared, ostracized, and threatened. Consider the following examples:

- A Harvard-educated attorney with AIDS was forced out of a job at a major Texas law firm. He said that to have AIDS is "like wearing the scarlet letter" (Rushing, 1995, p. 174).
- In White Plains, New York, a mailman refused to deliver mail to an AIDS task force office for 2 weeks because he feared he would catch the virus (Herek & Glunt, 1988).
- Three Florida brothers tested positive for HIV. Word spread. The boys' barber refused to cut their hair and the family's minister suggested they not attend weekly church services. Subsequently, the family's house was burned down (Herek & Glunt, 1988).
- A pilot reportedly said he wanted to throw Ron Doud off his plane when he learned that the New York-based interior designer had AIDS. When Doud arrived at his mother's home in Phoenix, medical center staff there were "very afraid to handle him." They simply placed his body in a plastic bag when he died (Altman, 1987, p. 62).

In fairness, these incidents occurred in the 1980s, when fear of AIDS was at an all-time high and knowledge of AIDS transmission had not diffused widely through American society. During the ensuing years, Americans have become more knowledgeable about how HIV is transmitted. They have also become more accepting of PWAs as they learned of the rich and textured lives led by individuals with HIV/AIDS, the loving care these persons have received from families, and the need to extend compassion to victims of a debilitating disease (Herek, 1997). Indeed, more than 75% of respondents to a national survey agreed that PWAs are unfairly persecuted (Herek, 1999). Even so, AIDS stigma remains a problem.

A significant minority of Americans favors coercive public policies, such as quarantining HIV-infected individuals, an option opposed by public health experts (Herek, 1997). PWAs have been evaluated more negatively than individuals suffering from other diseases, even by some health care professionals. Eight percent of the incidents of anti-gay harassment documented by a national gay and lesbian task force in 1994 concerned AIDS bias (Herek, 1997). The stigma associated with AIDS has even spread to those who volunteer to help PWAs. AIDS volunteers experience greater stigmatization than other volunteers in the health field, leading Mark Snyder and his colleagues (1999) to conclude that "AIDS volunteers are socially punished for their good deeds" (p. 1189).

What accounts for these findings? Why do people—including those who regard themselves as kind and intelligent—harbor negative attitudes toward those who contracted a biological virus? Are there rational reasons for these attitudes, or are they rooted in prejudice?

Explanations of AIDS Stigma

There is an obvious reason why people are reluctant to associate with PWAs. They are afraid that they will contract the disease. This is one reason why parents protested the decision to permit Ryan White, a hemophiliac child, to attend school in Kokomo, Indiana, when he was diagnosed with AIDS. Parents were nervous that Ryan would infect their own children. Even though some parents probably knew that AIDS cannot be transmitted through casual contact, they may have disregarded the information. In an age when experts are not all of one mind on medical issues and new evidence seems to contradict old facts, parents may have harbored an understandable fear that their children might contract AIDS through transmission routes that would only later be discovered.

Psychologists term this the *instrumental* basis of a negative attitude toward AIDS. According to this view, people stigmatize PWAs because they are afraid that they or loved ones will contract HIV through casual contact. (In fact, causal contact poses no risk because the skin contains an external protective layer that prevents HIV from entering the body's immune cells.) Facts notwithstanding, many people are afraid of being infected through contact with PWAs, and there is evidence that these fears can contribute to AIDS stigma (Bishop et al., 1991; Crandall, Glor, & Britt, 1997). Consider the feelings expressed by Jeanne Blake, a medical reporter for WBZ TV who was working on a story about the AIDS crisis in the inner city. Experiencing a sudden pang of guilt, Blake kissed John, a friend of hers who had AIDS, and then panicked.

> When I got home, a half hour later, I peeled off my jeans and tee shirt and jumped into the shower. The room was so hot. I could feel the virus in the air. I must have gotten infected! I kissed his hands right after he coughed! My husband, who had followed me into the room, stood watching me, dumbstruck. "I cannot believe what you're saying," he said. "You know you cannot get infected that way." That night I slept poorly, waking several times drenched with perspiration. "Night sweats. I am positive it's night sweats." My mind turned to my sexual past. "What if I am infected? What if I suffer like John has suffered? Who will take care of me?" The next morning I called an AIDS researcher whom I had interviewed. After I relayed the events of the night before, he said, "I understand your fear. I have gone through my own fears. I have been spit upon, phlegm has gotten in my eye, and on my mouth when patients coughed around me. But I am not infected and you didn't get infected last night either." (Goodgame, Blake, & Schwartz, 1992, pp. 306–307)

Thus, one reason people stigmatize—even shun—those who have AIDS is that they are afraid of contracting the virus. Some of this is understandable, an unfortunate but natural reaction to a strange and deadly disease. However, not all aspects of people's fears of PWAs are steeped in reasonable (if flawed) estimates of real-world consequences.

A less rational explanation for AIDS-related stigma is that it reflects a deep-seated belief in *a magical law of contagion* (Rozin, Markwith, & Nemeroff, 1992). According to this view, people, even in technologically advanced countries like the United States, adhere to a primitive belief that when two objects come into contact, they pass properties to each other and will continue from that point to influence each other. Like schoolgirls who are afraid of getting cooties from touching an unpopular student, grown-ups fear that if they come into contact with a person with AIDS they will magically get the virus.

Paul Rozin and his colleagues (1992) documented this phenomenon. In one portion of their experiment, they asked students to rate the pleasantness of wearing a sweater worn for 1 day by a man with AIDS. The sweater was described as having been washed after the man wore it. Subjects indicated it would be rather unpleasant to wear the sweater, even a full year after it had been worn only once by a man with AIDS. In reality, the sweater could not possibly transmit the AIDS virus.

There are several explanations for this finding, in addition to the one advanced by Rozin. Truth be told, many people would not wear a laundered sweater belonging to any stranger, let alone a stranger with AIDS. But some people appear to be less likely to wear a sweater that had been worn by a PWA (and then cleaned) than a sweater worn by a person without AIDS (Herek & Capitanio, 1999). Could it be that at some magical level of consciousness some of us fear that we will be contaminated by coming into casual contact with a PWA?

AIDS as a Social Symbol.   Like magical contagion, the third explanation for AIDS stigma emphasizes associations between AIDS and social objects. However, this view stresses the connection people make between AIDS and groups they don't like. As John Pryor and Glenn Reeder (1993) pointed out:

> HIV/AIDS may have acquired a symbolic meaning in our culture. As a symbol or a metaphor, it represents things like homosexual promiscuity, moral decadence, and the wrath of God for moral transgressions. . . . So, when people react negatively to someone with AIDS (or HIV), they may be expressing their feelings about the symbol. This analysis could explain why those strongly opposed to homosexuality react negatively to nonhomosexuals with HIV. Even the infected child bears the symbol of homosexual promiscuity. (p. 279)

More formally, Pryor and Reeder argue that we learn to represent people and ideas in certain ways in our heads. A person with AIDS (called a person node) is not a neutral entity but is connected with all sorts of other ideas and emotions that come to mind when we think about AIDS. AIDS (or HIV) may be associ-

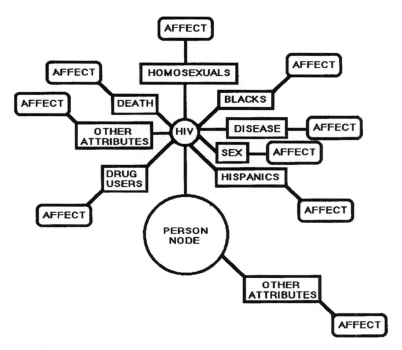

FIG. 7.1. An associative network representation of a person with HIV. From "Collective and individual representations of HIV/AIDS stigma" (p. 271), by J. B. Pryor and G. D. Reeder. In J. B. Pryor and G. D. Reeder (Eds.), *The Social Psychology of HIV Infection*, 1993, Hillsdale, NJ: Lawrence Erlbaum Associates.

ated in an individual's mind with homosexuals, drug users, minorities, promiscuous sex, even death. All of these entities are charged with emotion or affect. These emotions become powerfully associated with a person with AIDS (see Fig. 7.1). If someone thinks of HIV/AIDS as a disease involving homosexuality and despises homosexuals, then AIDS, homosexuality, and hate will mesh into a unified cognition and will come to mind when PWAs are discussed (Pryor, Reeder, & Landau, 1999).

Of course it can work the other way. You could have positive feelings about homosexuality. In this case, a PWA will call to mind positive sentiments, such as a person conducting an uplifting struggle against the forces of nature.

Unfortunately, for many people in the United States, homosexuality evokes negative sentiments. So does injection drug use. Thus, Pryor and Reeder make an interesting point when they argue that negative reactions to PWAs arise from the association of HIV with stigmatizing attributes.

There is empirical support for this view of AIDS stigma. Pryor and his colleagues (1989) asked students to imagine having a child in a class with a hemophiliac who was diagnosed with AIDS. Students who harbored negative attitudes toward homosexuality felt most negatively about their children interacting with a hemophiliac with AIDS. Notice that the person their child would encounter is not gay. Presumably, as George D. Bishop and his colleagues (1991) note, "AIDS evokes in people's minds the stigma associated with homosexuality and thus *anyone* with AIDS, even individuals who are demonstrably nonhomosexual, such as children who were infected with HIV through blood transfusions or female sexual partners of PWAs, comes to bear that stigma" (p. 1878).

Despite the fact that groups other than gay men are increasingly getting AIDS, many heterosexual Americans continue to link AIDS with homosexuality. In addition, a gay man who contracts AIDS through sex is blamed more for his infection than a heterosexual man or woman who became infected sexually (Herek & Capitanio, 1999). To be sure, even gay activists have criticized the gay community's conventional emphasis on hedonism (Rotello, 1997), with some coming close to blaming gay men for engaging in highly promiscuous unsafe sex. Nonetheless, it is illogical to blame gay men who contract AIDS sexually more than heterosexuals who contract AIDS through sex. The fact that many Americans do this suggests that AIDS-related stigma has roots in sexual prejudice.

Other biases also contribute to AIDS-related stigma. In the United States, negative attitudes toward injecting drug users play a role. People who hold more negative attitudes toward drug users also harbor more stigmatizing attitudes toward those who have AIDS (Capitanio & Herek, 1999). In Thailand, hostility toward prostitutes, many of whom are infected, contributes to AIDS stigma. In South Africa, women who contract HIV are blamed and beaten. Some are rejected by families and thrown out of their churches. "Many go to their graves with their secret, so great is the stigma," one reporter concluded (Daley, 1998, p. 1). This in turn has major consequences for African society. It discourages people from wanting to discover if they have AIDS, inhibits them from seeking health services, and increases the chances they will unwittingly spread the virus to others.

REDUCING AIDS STIGMA THROUGH PERSUASION

AIDS stigma is complex. It differs, depending on the society, the methods by which HIV is spread, values of a particular culture, and prejudices people harbor toward groups associated with the disease. People's attitudes toward PWAs also are complex. Some folks would never shake hands with a gay PWA, but harbor no prejudice toward gay people and may even have gay friends. For these people, AIDS stigma may reflect fear of getting infected or irrational feelings of magical contagion. Other people sympathize with the plight of those who lost loved ones to AIDS, but feel disgusted when thinking about an injecting drug user with AIDS. Other individuals may shy away from criticizing stigmatized groups in public to maintain a positive image. In the privacy of their living rooms, they may denounce gay men with AIDS, logging on to chat rooms that call gay men diseased or unclean.

Given the complexity of AIDS stigma, changing attitudes is not easy. Indeed, for those whose attitudes are rooted in a visceral hate of stigmatized groups, it is probably not possible to change attitudes at all. "Hate," as Andrew Sullivan (1999) poignantly observed, "will never disappear from human consciousness; in fact, it is probably, at some level, definitive of it" (p. 112). But for many others, change is possible. One of the themes of this book is that we can use persuasion to make things better for people if we understand theory and apply it sensitively and intelligently. So it is with AIDS stigma. In the United States, stigmatized attitudes toward PWAs have diminished in recent years (Herek, 1999), in part thanks to exposure to media information. But more can be done. Here are four suggestions:

First, persuaders should emphasize that HIV can be treated with drug therapies. Messages should stress that people can survive HIV infection (in varying degrees, of course). One of the reasons AIDS is stigmatizing is its connection with death. By disassociating AIDS from death, we can help reduce AIDS stigma in the same way that stigma associated with cancer has disappeared as chemotherapy has become commonplace.

Second, campaigns can humanize PWAs, showing how they cope with the disease and are living normal lives. Personal stories can be told. Individuals with AIDS can be transformed from victims to flesh-and-blood human beings. Messages could focus on a person with AIDS, telling audience members how this person is like them in more ways than they might have guessed. For example, we could listen as the PWA tells us how he works like the dickens to put a child through college, goes crazy when his baseball team wins the pennant, and gets depressed when he feels people are talking about him behind his back. Such messages, which could be tailored to audience segments through web sites, could point up the human aspect of AIDS and help the public frame AIDS as a virus affecting individuals, not social groups.

Communications like these are particularly important in Africa, where people have been killed by neighbors for revealing they are HIV-positive. However, change is coming to Africa and there is every reason to believe that communications can reduce AIDS stigma there. Consider that a man named Lucky Mazibuko, who is HIV-positive, was hired by a South African daily newspaper a couple of years ago to write a weekly column. "He wanted to show the nation that a black man could live with the human immunodeficiency virus and still hold his head high," a reporter noted. The column is titled "Just Call me Lucky" because, as Mazibuko notes, "I'm the luckiest man in the world" (Swarns, 1999, p. 1). To humanize PWAs, Mazibuko emphasizes that he is much like others who have the disease; at the same time he urges readers to make changes in their lives, such as using condoms and assuming responsibility for their sex lives.

A third way campaigns can reduce AIDS stigma is to stress the virtues of displaying compassion for PWAs. If, as Patricia Devine and her colleagues (1999) note, campaigns "are created in which tolerance for PWAs is portrayed as part of a positive social identity that is held by the majority (e.g., being a humanitarian), behavioral change could be facilitated in both the short- and long-term" (p. 1225). Gently using the self-confrontational strategy discussed in chapter 5, persuaders could encourage people to take note of the incongruence between their view of themselves as kind, decent people and their subtle prejudice toward PWAs. The dissonance might motivate self-criticism and attitude change.

A fourth approach, suggested recently by journalist Andrew Sullivan (1999), is to target attitudes of persons with AIDS, rather than everyone else. Sullivan suggests that PWAs loosen up and deflect prejudicial comments offered by people by considering their source of origin. He points out that:

> A hater cannot psychologically wound if a victim cannot psychologically be wounded. And that immunity to hurt can never be given; it can merely be achieved. The . . . epithet only strikes at someone's core if he lets it, if he allows the bigot's definition of him to be the final description of his life and his person— if somewhere in his heart of hearts, he believes the hateful slur to be true. . . . The only permanent rebuke to homophobia is not the enforcement of tolerance, but gay equanimity in the face of prejudice. . . . In this, as in so many other things, there is no solution to the problem. There is only a transcendence of it. (p. 113)

This is not to say that every verbal attack should be ignored, nor that physical abuse should be tolerated. They should be fought with tools of persuasion and the law, perhaps more than Sullivan suggested in this brief excerpt. However, Sullivan's iconoclastic approach is interesting because it empowers PWAs by reminding them that they can control how they respond to people's prejudices. It turns the problem around, and in so doing offers PWAs—and all targets of prejudice—a strategy for deflecting others' hate.

CONCLUSION

There is stigma associated with AIDS. People with AIDS bear a psychological mark that defines them as deviant or flawed in the eyes of too many people here and abroad. Although Americans in general have become more tolerant of PWAs, there are significant minorities of individuals who hate those with AIDS. Even as the media have publicized cases of celebrities who have become infected with HIV, there are large numbers of people who remain deeply unsettled at the thought of someone with AIDS and view PWAs as undesirable human beings.

People harbor stigmatizing attitudes for three reasons: First, they are afraid they will contract the virus if they come into contact with a person with AIDS; second, mythical views of contagion operate, convincing people that the HIV will be passed on to them if they encounter a PWA; and finally, AIDS calls to mind images of homosexuality, drug users, and minority groups, which, for many people, are tinged with negative affect.

Persuasive communication can reduce prejudice toward individuals with AIDS by humanizing PWAs. Messages can remind people that prejudice is not consistent with the values they place on tolerance and compassion for those who are struggling with disease.

On a larger level, it is important for PWAs to remain visible to the population. If those with AIDS retreat into their cocoons, it becomes easier for bigots to malign them, call them names, and transform them into objects rather than human beings. If those who have HIV/AIDS are out there, showing the world that they confront the virus in a Sisyphian way, pushing the rock up the hill each day after it tumbles down, they stand as testaments to the durability of the human spirit. By their own example, they humanize AIDS. They show that it is possible to do two things that appear inconsistent: contract a life-threatening disease and live an uplifting life.

References

Adelman, M. B. (1992). Healthy passions: Safer sex as play. In T. Edgar, M. A. Fitzpatrick, & V. S. Freimuth (Eds.), *AIDS: A communication perspective* (pp. 69–89). Hillsdale, NJ: Lawrence Erlbaum Associates.

Ajzen, I. (1991). The theory of planned behavior. *Organizational Behavior and Human Decision Processes, 50,* 179–211.

Ajzen, I., & Fishbein, M. (1980). *Understanding attitudes and predicting social behavior.* Englewood Cliffs, NJ: Prentice-Hall.

Alstead, M., Campsmith, M., Halley, C. S., Hartfield, K., Goldbaum, G., & Wood, R. W. (1999). Developing, implementing, and evaluating a condom promotion program targeting sexually active adolescents. *AIDS Education and Prevention, 11,* 497–512.

Altman, D. (1987). *AIDS in the mind of America.* Garden City, NY: Anchor.

Altman, L. K. (1999a, August 31). Focusing on prevention in fight against AIDS. *The New York Times,* p. D5.

Altman, L. K. (1999b, September 1). Much more AIDS in prisons than in general populations. *The New York Times,* p. A14.

Altman, L. K. (1999c, November 30). New book challenges theories of AIDS origins. *The New York Times,* pp. D1, D6.

Altman, L. K. (1998, November 24). Dismaying experts, HIV infections soar. *The New York Times,* p. D7.

Amaro, H. (1995). Love, sex, and power: Considering women's realities in HIV prevention. *American Psychologist, 50,* 437–447.

Ames, L. J., Atchinson, A. B., & Rose, D. T. (1995). Love, lust, and fear: Safer sex decision making among gay men. *Journal of Homosexuality, 30,* 53–73.

Ashery, R. S., Carlson, R. G., Flack, R. S., Siegal, H. A., & Wang, J. (1995). Female condom use among injection drug- and crack cocaine-using women. *American Journal of Public Health, 85,* 736–737.

Aspinwall, L. G., Kemeny, M. E., Taylor, S. E., Schneider, S. G., & Dudley, J. P. (1991). Psychosocial predictors of gay men's AIDS risk-reduction behavior. *Health Psychology, 10,* 432–444.

Bailey, W. A. (1995). The importance of HIV prevention programming to the lesbian and gay community. In G. M. Herek & B. Greene (Eds.), *AIDS, identity, and community: The HIV epidemic and lesbians and gay men* (pp. 210–225). Thousand Oaks, CA: Sage.

Bakker, A. B. (1999). Persuasive communication about AIDS prevention: Need for cognition determines the impact of message format. *AIDS Education and Prevention, 11,* 150- 162.

Bakker, A. B., Buunk, B. B., & Manstead, A. S. R. (1997). The moderating role of self-efficacy beliefs in the relationship between anticipated feelings of regret and condom use. *Journal of Applied Social Psychology, 27,* 2001–2014.

Bandura, A. (1977). Self-efficacy: Toward a unifying theory of behavioral change. *Psychological Review, 84,* 191–215.

Bandura, A. (1990). Perceived self-efficacy in the exercise of control over AIDS infection. *Evaluation and Program Planning, 13,* 9–17.

Bandura, A. (1992). A social cognitive approach to the exercise of control over AIDS infection. In R. J. DiClemente (Ed.), *Adolescents and AIDS: A generation in jeopardy* (pp. 89–116). Thousand Oaks, CA: Sage.

Bandura, A. (1994). Social cognitive theory and exercise of control over HIV infection. In R. DiClemente & J. L. Peterson (Eds.), *Preventing AIDS: Theories and methods of behavioral interventions* (pp. 25–59). New York: Plenum.

Bandura, A. (1995). Exercise of personal and collective efficacy in changing societies. In A. Bandura (Ed.), *Self-efficacy in changing societies* (pp. 1–45). New York: Cambridge University Press.

Bandura, A. (1998, August). *Swimming against the mainstream: Accenting the positive aspects of humanity.* Invited address presented at the annual convention of the American Psychological Association, San Francisco.

Barron, J. (1997, October 28). Officials link man to at least 10 girls infected with H. I. V. *The New York Times,* p. A19.

Basen-Engquist, K. (1992). Psychosocial predictors of "safe sex" behaviors in young adults. *AIDS Education and Prevention, 4,* 120–134.

Bauman, L. J., & Siegel, K. (1987). Misperception among gay men of the risk for AIDS associated with their sexual behavior. *Journal of Applied Social Psychology, 17,* 329–350.

Baxter, L. A., & Wilmot, W. W. (1985). Taboo topics in close relationships. *Journal of Social and Personal Relationships, 2,* 253–269.

Bayer, R. (1994). AIDS prevention and cultural sensitivity: Are they compatible? *American Journal of Public Health, 84,* 895–898.

Becker, M. H. (1974). The health belief model and personal health behavior. *Health Education Monographs, 2,* 324–508.

Becker, M. H., & Rosenstock, I. M. (1987). Comparing social learning theory and the health belief model. In W. B. Ward (Ed.), *Advances in health education and promotion* (Vol. 2, pp. 245–249). Greenwich, CT: JAI Press.

Belluck, P. (1998, October 12). In Small Town, U.S.A., AIDS presents new set of hardships. *The New York Times,* pp. A1, A13.

Berger, C. R. (1988). Planning, affect, and social action generation. In L. Donohew, H. E. Sypher, & E. T. Higgins (Eds.), *Communication, social cognition, and affect* (pp. 93–116). Hillsdale, NJ: Lawrence Erlbaum Associates.

Berger, C. R. (1997). Producing messages under uncertainty. In J. O. Greene (Ed.), *Message production: Advances in communication theory* (pp. 221–244). Mahwah, NJ: Lawrence Erlbaum Associates.

Berger, C. R., & Bell, R. A. (1988). Plans and the initiation of social relationships. *Human Communication Research, 15,* 217–235.

Binson, D., & Catania, J. A. (1998). Respondents' understanding of the words used in sexual behavior questions. *Public Opinion Quarterly, 62,* 190–208.

Bishop, G. D., Alva, A. L., Cantu, L., & Rittiman, T. K. (1991). Responses to persons with AIDS: Fear of contagion or stigma? *Journal of Applied Social Psychology, 21,* 1877–1888.

Blair, C., Ojakaa, D., Ochola, S. A., & Gogi, D. (1997). Barriers to behavior change: Results of focus group discussions conducted in a high HIV/AIDS incidence area of Kenya. In W. N. Elwood (Ed.), *Power in the blood: A handbook on AIDS, politics, and communication* (pp. 47–57). Mahwah, NJ: Lawrence Erlbaum Associates.

Bloom, B. R. (1998). The highest attainable standard: Ethical issues in AIDS vaccines. *Science, 279,* 186–188.

Bolton, R. (1992). AIDS and promiscuity: Muddles in the models. In R. Bolton & M. Singer (Eds.), *Rethinking AIDS prevention: Cultural approaches* (pp. 7–85). New York: Gordon & Breach.

Bowen, S. P., & Michal-Johnson, P. (1989). The crisis of communicating in relationships: Confronting the threat of AIDS. *AIDS & Public Policy Journal, 4,* 10–19.

Brafford, L. J., & Beck, K. H. (1991). Development and validation of a condom self-efficacy scale for college students. *Journal of American College Health, 39,* 219–225.

Brenders, D. A., & Garrett, L. (1993). Perceived control in the age of AIDS: A review of prevention information in academic, popular, and medical accounts. In S. C. Ratzan (Ed.), *AIDS: Effective health communication for the 90s* (pp. 113–140). Washington, DC: Taylor & Francis.

Brien, T. M., Thombs, D. L., Mahoney, C. A., & Wallnau, L. (1994). Dimensions of self-efficacy among three distinct groups of condom users. *Journal of American College Health, 42,* 167–174.

Brown, L. K., Lourie, K. J., Flanagan, P., & High, P. (1998). HIV-related attitudes and risk behavior of young adolescent mothers. *AIDS Education and Prevention, 10,* 565–573.

Brown, W. J., & Basil, M. D. (1995). Media celebrities and public health: Responses to "Magic" Johnson's HIV disclosure and its impact on AIDS risk and high-risk behaviors. *Health Communication, 7,* 345–370.

Bryan, A. D., Aiken, L. S., & West, S. G. (1997). Young women's condom use: The influence of acceptance of sexuality, control over the sexual encounter, and perceived susceptibility to common STDs. *Health Psychology, 16,* 468–479.

Bryan, A. D., Aiken, L. S., & West, S. G. (1999). The impact of males proposing condom use on perceptions of an initial sexual encounter. *Personality and Social Psychology Bulletin, 25,* 275–286.

Cameron, K. A., Witte, K., & Nzyuko, S. (1999). Perceptions of condoms and barriers to condom use along the Trans-Africa Highway in Kenya. In W. N. Elwood (Ed.), *Power in the blood: A handbook on AIDS, politics, and communication* (pp. 149–163). Mahwah, NJ: Lawrence Erlbaum Associates.

Capitanio, J. P., & Herek, G. M. (1999). AIDS-related stigma and attitudes toward injecting drug users among Black and White Americans. *American Behavioral Scientist, 42,* 1148–1161.

Carballo-Diéguez, A., & Dolezal, C. (1996). HIV risk behaviors and obstacles to condom use among Puerto Rican men in New York City who have sex with men. *American Journal of Public Health, 86,* 1619–1622.

Carmel, S. (1991). The health belief model in the research of AIDS-related preventive behavior. *Public Health Reviews, 18,* 73–85.

Carvajal, S. C., Garner, R. L., & Evans, R. I. (1998). Dispositional optimism as a protective factor in resisting HIV exposure in sexually active inner-city minority adolescents. *Journal of Applied Social Psychology, 28,* 2196–2211.

Catania, J. A., Chitwood, D. D., Gibson, D. R., & Coates, T. J. (1990). Methodological problems in AIDS behavioral research: Influences on measurement error and participation bias in studies of sexual behavior. *Psychological Bulletin, 108,* 339–362.

Catania, J. A., Coates, T. J., Kegeles, S. M., Fullilove, M. T., Peterson, J., Marin, B., Siegel, D., & Hulley, S. (1992). Condom use in multiethnic neighborhoods of San Francisco: The population-based AMEN (AIDS in multiethnic neighborhoods) study. *American Journal of Public Health, 82,* 284–287.

Catania, J. A., Kegeles, S. M., & Coates, T. J. (1990). Towards an understanding of risk behavior: An AIDS risk reduction model (ARRM). *Health Education Quarterly, 17,* 53–72.

Centers for Disease Control and Prevention (CDC). (1999a). *HIV/AIDS surveillance report, 11*(1), 3–42. Atlanta: U. S. Public Health Service.

Centers for Disease Control and Prevention. (1999b). *HIV/AIDS among Hispanics in the United States* [Online]. Available: http://www.cdc.gov

Centers for Disease Control and Prevention. (2000). *Sexual behaviors* [Online]. Available: http://www.cdc.gov

Chan, D. K-S., & Fishbein, M. (1993). Determinants of college women's intentions to tell their partners to use condoms. *Journal of Applied Social Psychology, 23,* 1455–1470.

Chay-Nemeth, C. (1998). Demystifying AIDS in Thailand: A dialectical analysis of the Thai sex industry. *Journal of Health Communication, 3,* 217–231.

Cline, R. J. W., & McKenzie, N. J. (1996). HIV/AIDS, women, and threads of discrimination: A tapestry of disenfranchisement. In E. Berlin Ray (Ed.), *Communication and disenfranchisement: Social health issues and implications* (pp. 365–386). Mahwah, NJ: Lawrence Erlbaum Associates.

Cline, R. J. W., Johnson, S. J., & Freeman, K. E. (1992). Talk among sexual partners about AIDS: Interpersonal communication for risk reduction or risk enhancement? *Health Communication, 4*, 39–56.

Coates, T. J. (1990). Strategies for modifying sexual behavior for primary and secondary prevention of HIV disease. *Journal of Consulting and Clinical Psychology, 58*, 57–69.

Cochran, S. D., & Mays, V. M. (1990). Sex, lies, and HIV [Letter to the Editor]. *The New England Journal of Medicine, 322*, 774–775.

Cochran, S. D., & Mays, V. M. (1993). Applying social psychological models to predicting HIV-related sexual risk behaviors among African Americans. *Journal of Black Psychology, 19*, 142–154.

Connors, M. (1992). Risk perception, risk taking and risk management among intravenous drug users: Implications for AIDS prevention. *Social Science and Medicine, 34*, 591–601.

Connors, M. (1996). Sex, drugs, and structural violence. In P. Farmer, M. Connors, & J. Simmons (Eds.), *Women, poverty and AIDS: Sex, drugs, and structural violence* (pp. 91–123). Monroe, ME: Common Courage Press.

Corby, N. H., Jamner, M., & Wolitski, R. J. (1996). Using the theory of planned behavior to predict intention to use condoms among male and female injecting drug users. *Journal of Applied Social Psychology, 26*, 52–75.

Crandall, C. S., Glor, J., & Britt, T. W. (1997). AIDS-related stigmatization: Instrumental and symbolic attitudes. *Journal of Applied Social Psychology, 27*, 95–123.

Crawford, A. M. (1996). Stigma associated with AIDS: A meta-analysis. *Journal of Applied Social Psychology, 26*, 398–416.

Curtius, M. (1999, September 12). New tactics debated in war on AIDS. *The Plain Dealer*, p. 10-A.

Dahl, D. W., Gorn, G. J., & Weinberg, C. B. (1997). Marketing, safer sex, and condom acquisition. In M. E. Goldberg, M. Fishbein, & S. E. Middlestadt (Eds.), *Social marketing: Theoretical and practical perspectives* (pp. 169–185). Mahwah, NJ: Lawrence Erlbaum Associates.

Daley, S. (1998, December 4). AIDS is everywhere, but the Africans look away. *The New York Times*, pp. A1, A12.

Dalton, H. L. (1989). AIDS in blackface. *Daedelus, 118, 3*, 205–227.

Davis, D. (2000, March 15). Life in the shadow of death. *The Plain Dealer*, pp. 1-A, 16-A, 17-A.

Daum, M. (1996, January 21). Safe-sex lies. *The New York Times Magazine*, pp. 32–33.

Dearing, J. W., Larson, R. S., Randall, L. M., & Pope, R. S. (1998). Local reinvention of the CDC HIV prevention community planning initiative. *Journal of Community Health, 23*, 113–126.

Dearing, J. W., Meyer, G., & Rogers, E. M. (1994). Diffusion theory and HIV risk behavior change. In R. J. DiClemente & J. L. Peterson (Eds.), *Preventing AIDS: Theories and methods of behavioral interventions* (pp. 79–93). New York: Plenum.

Dearing, J. W., & Rogers, E. M. (1992). AIDS and the media agenda. In T. Edgar, M. A. Fitzpatrick, & V. S. Freimuth (Eds.), *AIDS: A communication perspective* (pp. 173–194). Hillsdale, NJ: Lawrence Erlbaum Associates.

Dearing, J. W., Rogers, E. M., Meyer, G., Casey, M. K., Rao, N., Campo, S., & Henderson, G. M. (1996). Social marketing and diffusion-based strategies for communicating with unique populations: HIV prevention in San Francisco. *Journal of Health Communication, 1*, 343–363.

De Bro, S. C., Campbell, S. M., & Peplau, L. A. (1994). Influencing a partner to use a condom: A college student perspective. *Psychology of Women Quarterly, 18*, 165–182.

DeJong, W., & Winsten, J. A. (1992). The strategic use of the broadcast media for AIDS prevention: Current limits and future directions. In J. Sepulveda, H. Fineberg, & J. Mann (Eds.), *AIDS prevention through education: A world view* (pp. 255–272). New York: Oxford University Press.

Delaporte, F. (1986). *Disease and civilization: The cholera in Paris, 1832*. Cambridge, Mass: MIT Press.

Derrida, J. (1976). *Of grammatology*. Baltimore: Johns Hopkins University Press.

Devine, P. G., Plant, E. A., & Harrison, K. (1999). The problem of "us" versus "them" and AIDS stigma. *American Behavioral Scientist, 42*, 1212–1228.

Díaz, R. M. (1997). Latino gay men and psychocultural barriers to AIDS prevention. In M. P. Levine, P. M. Nardi, & J. H. Gagnon (Eds.), *In changing times: Gay men and lesbians encounter HIV/AIDS* (pp. 221–244). Chicago: University of Chicago Press.

Díaz, R. M. (1998). *Latino gay men and HIV: Culture, sexuality, and risk behavior.* New York: Routledge.

DiClemente, R. J. (1992a). (Ed.) *Adolescents and AIDS: A generation in jeopardy.* Thousand Oaks, CA: Sage.

DiClemente, R. J. (1992b). Psychosocial determinants of condom use among adolescents. In R. J. DiClemente (Ed.), *Adolescents and AIDS: A generation in jeopardy* (pp. 34–51). Thousand Oaks, CA: Sage.

Donovan, M. C. (1999). A tough sell: The political logic of federal needle-exchange policy. In W. N. Elwood (Ed.), *Power in the blood: A handbook on AIDS, politics, and communication* (pp. 353–368). Mahwah, NJ: Lawrence Erlbaum Associates.

Dostoevsky, F. (1960). *Notes from underground & The grand inquisitor.* New York: Dutton.

Duck, J. M., Terry, D. J., & Hogg, M. A. (1995). The perceived influence of AIDS advertising: Third-person effects in the context of positive media content. *Basic and Applied Social Psychology, 17,* 305–325.

Edgar, T. (1992). A compliance-based approach to the study of condom use. In T. Edgar, M. A. Fitzpatrick, & V. S. Freimuth (Eds.), *AIDS: A communication perspective* (pp. 47–67). Hillsdale, NJ: Lawrence Erlbaum Associates.

Edgar, T., & Fitzpatrick, M. A. (1988). Compliance-gaining in relational interaction: When your life depends on it. *Southern Speech Communication Journal, 53,* 385–405.

Edgar, T., & Fitzpatrick, M. A. (1993). Expectations for sexual interaction: A cognitive test of the sequencing of sexual communication behaviors. *Health Communication, 4,* 239–261.

Edgar, T., Freimuth, V. S., & Hammond, S. L. (1988). Communicating the AIDS risk to college students: The problem of motivating change. *Health Education Research, 3,* 59–65.

Edgar, T., Freimuth, V. S., Hammond, S. L., McDonald, D. A., & Fink, E. L. (1992). Strategic sexual communication: Condom use resistance and response. *Health Communication, 4,* 83–104.

Ekstrand, M. L., & Coates, T. J. (1990). Maintenance of safer sexual behaviors and predictors of risky sex: The San Francisco men's health study. *American Journal of Public Health, 80,* 973–977.

El-Bassel, N., Krishnan, S. P., Schilling, R. F., Witte, S., & Gilbert L. (1998). Acceptability of the female condom among STD clinic patients. *AIDS Education and Prevention, 10,* 465–480.

Elkins, D. B., Dole, L. R., Maticka-Tyndale, E., & Stam, K. R. (1998). Relaying the message of safer sex: Condom races for community-based skills training. *Health Education Research, 13,* 357–370.

Elwood, W. N., & Williams, M. L. (1999). The politics of silence: Communicative rules and HIV prevention issues in gay male bathhouses. In W. N. Elwood (Ed.), *Power in the blood: A handbook on AIDS, politics, and communication* (pp. 121–132). Mahwah, NJ: Lawrence Erlbaum Associates.

Emenike, I. (1997). Sexual abstinence: A viable option for young adolescents in HIV/AIDS prevention. In D. C. Umeh (Ed.), *Confronting the AIDS epidemic: Cross-cultural perspectives on HIV/AIDS education* (pp. 317–327). Trenton, NJ: Africa World Press.

Etzioni, A. (Ed.). (1998). *The essential communitarian reader.* Lanham, MD: Rowman & Littlefield.

Farmer, P. (1996). Women, poverty, and AIDS. In P. Farmer, M. Connors, & J. Simmons (Eds.), *Women, poverty and AIDS: Sex, drugs, and structural violence* (pp. 3–38). Monroe, ME: Common Courage Press.

Fee, E., & Fox, D. M. (1992). Introduction: The contemporary historiography of AIDS. In E. Fee & D. M. Fox (Eds.), *AIDS: The making of a chronic disease* (pp. 1–19). Berkeley, CA: University of California Press.

Fishbein, M. (1996). Great expectations, or do we ask too much from community-level interventions? *American Journal of Public Health, 86,* 1075–1076.

Fishbein, M., & Ajzen, I. (1975). *Belief, attitude, intention and behavior: An introduction to theory and research.* Reading, MA: Addison-Wesley.

Fishbein, M., Chan, D. K-S., O'Reilly, K., Schnell, D., Wood, R., Beeker, C., & Cohn, D. (1992). Attitudinal and normative factors as determinants of gay men's intentions to perform AIDS-related sexual behaviors: A multisite analysis. *Journal of Applied Social Psychology, 22,* 999–1011.

Fishbein, M., Guenther-Grey, C., Johnson, W., Wolitski, R. J., McAlister, A., Rietmeijer, C. A., & O'Reilly, K. O. (1997). Using a theory-based community intervention to reduce AIDS risk behaviors: The CDC's AIDS community demonstration projects. In M. E. Goldberg, M. Fishbein, & S. E. Middlestadt (Eds.), *Social marketing: Theoretical and practical perspectives* (pp. 123–146). Mahwah, NJ: Lawrence Erlbaum Associates.

Fishbein, M. & Guinan, M. (1996). Behavioral science and public health: A necessary partnership for HIV prevention. *Public Health Reports, 111*(Suppl. 1), 5–10.

Fishbein, M., & Middlestadt, S. E. (1989). Using the theory of reasoned action as a framework for understanding and changing AIDS-related behaviors. In V. M. Mays, G. W. Albee, & S. F Schneider (Eds.), *Primary prevention of AIDS: Psychological approaches* (pp. 93–110). Thousand Oaks, CA: Sage.

Fisher, J. D., & Fisher, W. A. (1996). The information-motivation-behavioral skills model of AIDS risk behavior change: Empirical support and application. In S. Oskamp & S. C. Thompson (Eds.), *Understanding and preventing HIV risk behavior: Safe sex and drug use* (pp. 100–127). Thousand Oaks, CA: Sage.

Fisher, J. D., Misovich, S. J., & Fisher, W. A. (1992). Impact of perceived social norms on adolescents' AIDS-risk behavior and prevention. In R. J. DiClemente (Ed.), *Adolescents and AIDS: A generation in jeopardy* (pp. 117–136). Thousand Oaks, CA: Sage.

Fisher, W. A., & Fisher, J. D. (1993). A general social psychological model for changing AIDS risk behavior. In J. B. Pryor & G. D. Reeder (Eds.), *The social psychology of HIV infection* (pp. 127–153). Hillsdale, NJ: Lawrence Erlbaum Associates.

Flora, J. A., Schooler, C., & Pierson, R. M. (1997). Effective health promotion among communities of color: The potential of social marketing. In M. E. Goldberg, M. Fishbein, & S. E. Middlestadt (Eds.), *Social marketing: Theoretical and practical perspectives* (pp. 353–373). Mahwah, NJ: Lawrence Erlbaum Associates.

Freimuth, V. S., Edgar, T., & Hammond, S. L. (1987). College students' awareness and interpretation of the AIDS risk. *Science, Technology, and Human Values, 12,* 37–40.

Fullilove, M. T., & Fullilove, R. E., III. (1999). Stigma as an obstacle to AIDS action: The case of the African American community. *American Behavioral Scientist, 42,* 1117–1129.

Fullilove, R. E., III. (1995). Community disintegration and public health: A case study of New York City. In *Assessing the social and behavioral science base for HIV/AIDS prevention and intervention: Workshop summary* (pp. 93–116). Washington, DC: National Academy Press.

Fumento, M. (1990). *The myth of heterosexual AIDS.* New York: Basic Books.

Galligan, R. F., & Terry, D. J. (1993). Romantic ideals, fear of negative implications, and the practice of safe sex. *Journal of Applied Social Psychology, 23,* 1685–1711.

Gerrard, M., Gibbons, F. X., & Bushman, B. J. (1996). Relation between perceived vulnerability to HIV and precautionary sexual behavior. *Psychological Bulletin, 119,* 390–409.

Giles, H., & Smith, P. M. (1979). Accommodation theory: Optimal levels of convergence. In H. Giles & R. N. St. Clair (Eds.), *Language and social psychology* (pp. 45–65). Baltimore: University Park Press.

Gillespie, C. C. (1997). Women's HIV risk reduction efforts and traditional models of health behavior: A review and critique. *Women's Health: Research on Gender, Behavior, and Policy, 3,* 1–30.

Gold, R. S., & Skinner, M. J. (1992). Situational factors and thought processes associated with unprotected intercourse in young gay men. *AIDS, 6,* 1021–1030.

Goldenberg, J. M., Pyszczynski, T., Johnson, K. D., Greenberg, J., & Solomon, S. (1999). The appeal of tragedy: A terror management perspective. *Media Psychology, 1,* 313–329.

Goldman, J. A., & Harlow, L. L. (1993). Self-perception variables that mediate AIDS-preventive behavior in college students. *Health Psychology, 12,* 489–498.

Goodgame, T., Blake, J., & Schwartz, G. (1992), Television's response to the AIDS crisis: One company's experience. In J. Sepulveda, H. Fineberg, & J. Mann (Eds.), *AIDS prevention through education: A world view* (pp. 297–319). New York: Oxford University Press.

Gordon, C. M., Carey, M. P., & Carey, K. B. (1997). Effects of a drinking event on behavioral skills and condom attitudes in men: Implications for HIV risk from a controlled experiment. *Health Psychology, 16,* 490–495.

Green, F. (1999, May 5–11). Cocktail hangover. *Cleveland Free Times,* pp. 20–24.

Green, J. (1996, September 15). Flirting with suicide. *The New York Times Magazine,* pp. 38–45, 54–55, 84–85.

Greenberg, B. S. & Busselle, R. W. (1996). Soap operas and sexual activity: A decade later. *Journal of Communication, 46*(4), 153–160.

Guenther-Grey, C., Noroian, D., Fonseka, J., & Higgins, D. (1996). Developing community networks to deliver HIV prevention interventions. *Public Health Reports, 110*(Suppl. 1), 41–49.

Guttman, N. (1997). Beyond strategic research: A value-centered approach to health communication interventions. *Communication Theory, 7,* 95–124.

Hage, J. (1972). *Techniques and problems of theory construction in sociology.* New York: Wiley.

Hammer, J. C., Fisher, J. D., Fitzergald, P., & Fisher, W. A. (1996). When two heads aren't better than one: AIDS risk behavior in college-age couples. *Journal of Applied Social Psychology, 26,* 375–397.

Hays, R. B., Kegeles, S. M., & Coates, T. J. (1990). High HIV risk-taking among young gay men. *AIDS, 4,* 901–907.

Heckman, T. G., Kelly, J. A., Sikkema, K. J., Roffman, R. R., Solomon, L. J., Winett, R. A., Stevenson, L. Y., Perry, M. J., Norman, A. D., & Desiderato, L. J. (1995). Differences in HIV risk characteristics between bisexual and exclusively gay men. *AIDS Education and Prevention, 7,* 504–512.

Helman, C. G. (1990). *Culture, health and illness* (2nd ed.). London: Wright and Sons.

Helweg-Larsen, M., & Collins, B. E. (1994). The UCLA multidimensional condom attitudes scale: Documenting the complex determinants of condom use in college students. *Health Psychology, 13,* 224–237.

Herek, G. M. (1997). The HIV epidemic and public attitudes toward lesbians and gay men. In M. P. Levine, P. M. Nardi, & J. H. Gagnon (Eds.), *In changing times: Gay men and lesbians encounter HIV/AIDS* (pp. 191–218). Chicago: University of Chicago Press.

Herek, G. M. (1999). AIDS and stigma. *American Behavioral Scientist, 42,* 1106–1116.

Herek, G. M., & Capitanio, J. P. (1999). AIDS stigma and sexual prejudice. *American Behavioral Scientist, 42,* 1130–1147.

Herek, G. M., & Glunt, E. K. (1988). An epidemic of stigma: Public reactions to AIDS. *American Psychologist, 43,* 886–891.

Hingson, R. W., Strunin, L., Berlin, B. M., & Heeren, T. (1990). Beliefs about AIDS, use of alcohol and drugs, and unprotected sex among Massachusetts adolescents. *American Journal of Public Health, 80,* 295–299.

Hobfoll, S. E., Jackson, A. P., Lavin, J., Britton, P. J., & Shepherd, J. B. (1993). Safer sex knowledge, behavior, and attitudes of inner-city women. *Health Psychology, 12,* 481–488.

Jemmott, J. B., III. (1996). Social psychological influences on HIV risk behavior among African American youth. In S. Oskamp & S. C. Thompson (Eds.), *Understanding and preventing HIV risk behavior: Safer sex and drug use* (pp. 131–156). Thousand Oaks, CA: Sage.

Jemmott, J. B., III., Jemmott, L. S., Spears, H., Hewitt, N., & Cruz-Collins, M. (1992). Self-efficacy, hedonistic expectancies, and condom-use intentions among inner-city Black adolescent women: A social cognitive approach to AIDS risk behavior. *Journal of Adolescent Health, 13,* 512–519.

Jemmott, J. B., III, & Jones, J. M. (1993). Social psychology and AIDS among ethnic minority individuals: Risk behaviors and strategies for changing them. In J. B. Pryor & G. D. Reeder (Eds.), *The social psychology of HIV infection* (pp. 183–224). Hillsdale, NJ: Lawrence Erlbaum Associates.

Jemmott, L. S., Catan, V., Nyamathi, A., & Anastasia, J. (1995). African American women and HIV-risk-reduction issues. In A. O'Leary & L. S. Jemmott (Eds.), *Women at risk: Issues in the primary prevention of AIDS* (pp. 131–157). New York: Plenum.

Jemmott, L. S., & Jemmott, J. B., III. (1991). Applying the theory of reasoned action to AIDS risk behavior: Condom use among Black women. *Nursing Research, 40,* 228–234.

Jemmott, L. S., & Jemmott, J. B., III. (1992). Increasing condom-use intentions among sexually active Black adolescent women. *Nursing Research, 41,* 273–279.

Joffe, H., & Dockrell, J. E. (1995). Safer sex: Lessons from the male sex industry. *Journal of Community & Applied Social Psychology, 5,* 333–346.

Johnson, E. H. (1993). *Risky sexual behaviors among African-Americans.* Westport, CT: Praeger.

Jones, E. E., Farina, A., Hastorf, A. H., Markus, H., Miller, D. T., & Scott, R. A. (1984). *Social stigma: The psychology of marked relationships.* New York: W. H. Freeman.

Kalichman, S. C. (1994). Magic Johnson and public attitudes toward AIDS: A review of empirical findings. *AIDS Education and Prevention, 6,* 542–557.

Kalichman, S. C. (1996). *Answering your questions about AIDS.* Washington, DC: American Psychological Association.

Kalichman, S. C. (1998). *Preventing AIDS: A sourcebook for behavioral interventions.* Mahwah, NJ: Lawrence Erlbaum Associates.

Kalichman, S. C., & Coley, B. (1995). Context framing to enhance HIV-antibody-testing messages targeted to African American women. *Health Psychology, 14,* 247–254.

Kalichman, S. C., Greenberg, J., & Abel, G. G. (1997). HIV-seropositive men who engage in high-risk sexual behavior: Psychological characteristics and implications for prevention. *AIDS Care, 9,* 441–450.

Kalichman, S. C., Heckman, T., & Kelly, J. A. (1996). Sensation-seeking, substance use, and HIV-AIDS risk behavior: Directional relationships among gay men. *Archives of Sexual Behavior, 25,* 141–154.

Kalichman, S. C., Kelly, J. A., & Rompa, D. (1997). Continued high-risk sex among HIV seropositive gay and bisexual men seeking HIV prevention services. *Health Psychology, 16,* 369–373.

Kaplan, B. J., & Shayne, V. T. (1993). Unsafe sex: Decision-making biases and heuristics. *AIDS Education and Prevention, 5,* 294–301.

Katz, D. (1960). The functional approach to the study of attitudes. *Public Opinion Quarterly, 24,* 163–204.

Kegeles, S. M., Hays, R. B., & Coates, T. J. (1996). The Mpowerment Project: A community-level HIV prevention intervention for young gay men. *American Journal of Public Health, 86,* 1129–1136.

Kellar-Guenther, Y. (1999). The power of romance: Changing the focus of AIDS education messages. In W. N. Elwood (Ed.), *Power in the blood: A handbook on AIDS, politics, and communication* (pp. 215–229). Mahwah, NJ: Lawrence Erlbaum Associates.

Kelly, J. A. (1995). *Changing HIV risk behavior: Practical strategies.* New York: Guilford.

Kelly, J. A., Murphy, D., Sikkema, K., McAuliffe, T., Roffman, R., Solomon, L., Winett, R., & Kalichman, S. C. (1997). Outcomes of a randomized controlled community-level HIV prevention intervention: Effects on behavior among at-risk gay men in small U.S. cities. *Lancet, 350,* 1500–1505.

Kelly, J. A., Murphy, D. A., Washington, C. D., Wilson, T. S., Koob, J. J., Davis, D. R., Ledezma, G., & Davantes, B. (1994). The effects of HIV/AIDS intervention groups for high-risk women in urban clinics. *American Journal of Public Health, 84,* 1918–1922.

Kelly, J. A., St. Lawrence, J. S., Diaz, Y. E., Stevenson, L. Y., Hauth, A. C., Brasfield, T. L., Kalichman, S. C., Smith, J. E., & Andrew, M. E. (1991). HIV risk behavior reduction following intervention with key opinion leaders of population: An experimental analysis. *American Journal of Public Health, 81,* 168–171.

Kelly, J. A., St. Lawrence, J. S., Hood, H. V., & Brasfield, T. L. (1989). Behavioral intervention to reduce AIDS risk activities. *Journal of Consulting and Clinical Psychology, 57,* 60–67.

Kelman, H. C. (1958). Compliance, identification, and internalization: Three processes of attitude change. *Journal of Conflict Resolution, 2,* 51–60.

Kernan, J. B., & Domzal, T. J. (1997). Hippocrates to Hermes: The postmodern turn in public health advertising. In M. E. Goldberg, M. Fishbein, & S. E. Middlestadt (Eds.), *Social marketing: Theoretical and practical perspectives* (pp. 387–416). Mahwah, NJ: Lawrence Erlbaum Associates.

Kinsella, J. (1988). *Covering the plague: AIDS and the American media.* New Brunswick, NJ: Rutgers University Press.

Kirsch, I. (1995). Self-efficacy and outcome expectancy: A concluding commentary. In J. E. Maddux (Ed.), *Self-efficacy, adaptation, and adjustment: Theory, research, and application* (pp. 331–345). New York: Plenum.

Krauss, B. J., Wolitski, R. J., Tross, S., Corby, N. H., & Fishbein, M. (1999). Getting the message: HIV information sources of women who have sex with injecting drug users—A two-site study. *Applied Psychology: An International Review, 48,* 153–173.

Lamptey, P., & Weir, S. (1992). Targeted AIDS intervention programs in Africa. In J. Sepulveda, H. Fineberg, & J. Mann (Eds.), *AIDS prevention through education: A world view* (pp. 145–174). New York: Oxford University Press.

Landers, A. (1998, December 28). Safe sex needs to be taught at an early age. *The New Jersey Star-Ledger,* p. 29.

Leeper, M. A. (1990). Preliminary evaluation of reality™, a condom for women. *AIDS Care, 2,* 287–290.

Leviton, L. C. (1989). Theoretical foundations of AIDS-prevention programs. In R. O. Valdiserri (Ed.), *Preventing AIDS: The design of effective programs* (pp. 42–90). New Brunswick, NJ: Rutgers University Press.

Lipsky, D. (1995, March 23). Latex generation: Sex on campus! *Rolling Stone,* pp. 80–86, 114.

Logan, T. K., Leukefeld, C., & Farabee, D. (1998). Sexual and drug use behaviors among women crack users: Implications for prevention. *AIDS Education and Prevention, 10,* 327–340.

MacDonald, T. K., Zanna, M. P., & Fong, G. T. (1996). Why common sense goes out the window: Effects of alcohol on intentions to use condoms. *Personality and Social Psychology Bulletin, 22,* 763–775.

Maibach, E. W., & Cotton, D. (1995). Moving people to behavior change: A staged social cognitive approach to message design. In E. Maibach & R. L. Parrott (Eds.), *Designing health messages: Approaches from communication theory and public health practice* (pp. 41–64). Thousand Oaks, CA: Sage.

Maibach, E., & Flora, J. A. (1993). Symbolic modeling and cognitive rehearsal: Using video to promote AIDS prevention self-efficacy. *Communication Research, 20,* 517–545.

Maibach, E. W., Kreps, G. L., & Bonaguro, E. W. (1993). Developing strategic communication campaigns for HIV/AIDS prevention. In S. Ratzan (Ed.), *AIDS: Effective health communication for the 90s* (pp. 15–35). Washington, DC: Taylor & Francis.

Marin, B. V., Tschann, J. M., Gomez, C. A., & Gregorich. S. (1998). Self-efficacy to use condoms in unmarried Latino adults. *American Journal of Community Psychology, 26,* 53–71.

Mattson, M. (1999). Toward a reconceptualization of communication cues to action in the health belief model: HIV test counseling. *Communication Monographs, 66,* 240–265.

Mays, V. M., & Cochran, S. D. (1988). Issues in the perception of AIDS risk and risk reduction activities by Black and Hispanic/Latina women. *American Psychologist, 43,* 949–957.

Mays, V. M., & Cochran, S. D. (1993). Ethnic and gender differences in beliefs about sex partner questioning to reduce HIV risk. *Journal of Adolescent Research, 8,* 77–88.

Mays, V. M, & Cochran, S. D. (1995). HIV/AIDS in the African-American community: Changing concerns, changing behaviors. In M. Stein & A. Baum (Eds.), *Chronic diseases* (pp. 259–272). Hillsdale, NJ: Lawrence Erlbaum Associates.

McGuire, W. J. (1985). Attitudes and attitude change. In G. Lindzey & E. Aronson (Eds.), *Handbook of social psychology* (3rd ed., Vol. 2, pp. 233–346). New York: Random House.

McGuire, W. J. (1989). Theoretical foundations of campaigns. In R. E. Rice & C. K. Atkin (Eds.), *Public communication campaigns* (2nd ed., pp. 43–65). Thousand Oaks, CA: Sage.

McKirnan, D. J., Ostrow, D. G., & Hope, B. (1996). Sex, drugs and escape: A psychological model of HIV-risk sexual behaviors. *AIDS Care, 8,* 655–669.

McKusick, L., Coates, T. J., Morin, S. F., Pollack, L., & Hoff, C. (1990). Longitudinal predictors of reductions in unprotected anal intercourse among gay men in San Francisco: The AIDS Behavioral Research Project. *American Journal of Public Health, 80,* 978–983.

McLaurin, P. (1995). An examination of the effect of culture on pro-social messages directed at African-American at-risk youth. *Communication Monographs, 62,* 301–326.

McNeil, D. G., Jr. (1999, July 24). Condoms for women gain approval among Africans. *The New York Times,* pp. 1, A6.

Metts, S., & Fitzpatrick, M. A. (1992). Thinking about safer sex: The risky business of "know your partner" advice. In T. Edgar, M. A. Fitzpatrick, & V. S. Freimuth (Eds.), *AIDS: A communication perspective* (pp. 1–19). Hillsdale, NJ: Lawrence Erlbaum Associates.

Metts, S., & Spitzberg, B. H. (1996). Sexual communication in interpersonal contexts: A script-based approach. In B. R. Burleson (Ed.), *Communication yearbook 19* (pp. 49–91). Thousand Oaks, CA: Sage.

Michal-Johnson, P., & Perlmutter Bowen, S. (1992). The place of culture in HIV education. In T. Edgar, M. A. Fitzpatrick, & V. S. Freimuth (Eds.), *AIDS: A communication perspective* (pp. 147–172). Hillsdale, NJ: Lawrence Erlbaum Associates.

Mickler, S. E. (1993). Perceptions of vulnerability: Impact on AIDS-preventive behavior among college students. *AIDS Education and Prevention, 5,* 43–53.

Middlestadt, S. E., Schechter, C., Peyton J., & Tjugum, B. (1997). Community involvement in health planning: Lessons learned from practicing social marketing in a context of community control, participation, and ownership. In M. E. Goldberg, M. Fishbein, & S. E. Middlestadt (Eds.), *Social marketing: Theoretical and practical perspectives* (pp. 291–311). Mahwah, NJ: Lawrence Erlbaum Associates.

Miller, J. B.(1986). *Toward a new psychology of women* (2nd ed.). Boston: Beacon Press.

Miller, L. C., Bettencourt, B. A., De Bro, S. C., & Hoffman, V. (1993). Negotiating safer sex: Interpersonal dynamics. In J. B. Pryor & G. D. Reeder (Eds.), *The social psychology of HIV infection* (pp. 85–123). Hillsdale, NJ: Lawrence Erlbaum Associates.

Mitchell, J. L., Thompson, R., Carrington, B. W., Namerow, P. B., Brown, L., Loftman, P. O., & Williams, S. B. (1997). AIDS in the Black/African-American community: A central Harlem experience. In D. C. Umeh (Ed.), *Confronting the AIDS epidemic: Cross-cultural perspectives on HIV/ AIDS education* (pp. 267–298). Trenton, NJ: Africa World Press.

Morisky, D. E., & Coan, D. L. (1998). Asia—The new epidemic zone for HIV/AIDS. *Journal of Health Communication, 3,* 185–191.

Morokoff, P. J., Mays, V. M., & Coons, H. L. (1997). HIV infection and AIDS. In S. J. Gallant, G. Puryear Keita, & R. Royak-Schaler (Eds.), *Health care for women: Psychological, social, and behavioral influences* (pp. 273–293). Washington, DC: American Psychological Association.

Morris, K. A., & Swann, W. B., Jr. (1996). Denial and the AIDS crisis: On wishing away the threat of AIDS. In S. Oskamp & S. C. Thompson (Eds.), *Understanding and preventing HIV risk behavior: Safer sex and drug use* (pp. 57–79). Thousand Oaks, CA: Sage.

Morse, S. S. (1992). AIDS and beyond: Defining the rules for viral traffic. In E. Fee & D. M. Fox (Eds.), *AIDS: The making of a chronic disease* (pp. 23–48). Berkeley, CA: University of California Press.

Moskowitz, J. T., Binson, D., & Catania, J. A. (1997). The association between Magic Johnson's HIV serostatus disclosure and condom use in at-risk respondents. *Journal of Sex Research, 34,* 154–160.

Myrick, R. (1998). In search of cultural sensitivity and inclusiveness: Communication strategies used in rural HIV prevention campaigns designed for African Americans. *Health Communication, 10,* 65–85.

Nathanson, N., & Auerbach, J. D. (1999). Confronting the HIV pandemic, *Science, 284,* 1619.

Needle, R. H., Coyle, S. L., Normand, J., Lambert, E., & Cesari, H. (1998). HIV prevention with drug-using populations—Current status and future prospects: Introduction and overview. *Public Health Reports, 113*(Suppl. 1), 4–18.

Netter, T. W. (1992). The media and AIDS: A global perspective. In J. Sepulveda, H. Fineberg, & J. Mann (Eds.), *AIDS prevention through education: A world view* (pp. 241–253). New York: Oxford University Press.

Nieves, E. (1999a, May 29). San Francisco is urged to allow secluded sex in bathhouses. *The New York Times,* p. A9.

Nieves, E. (1999b, August 25). Privacy questions raised in cases of syphilis linked to chat room. *The New York Times,* pp. 1, A16.

NIMH Multisite HIV Prevention Trial Group. (1998). The NIMH multisite HIV prevention trial: Reducing HIV sexual risk behavior. *Science, 280,* 1889–1894.

Norman, D. A. (1988). *The psychology of everyday things.* New York: Basic Books.

Nyakabwa, K. (1997). Uganda and the challenge of AIDS. In D. C. Umeh (Ed.), *Confronting the AIDS epidemic: Cross-cultural perspectives on HIV/AIDS education* (pp. 27–38). Trenton, NJ: Africa World Press.

Nyamathi, A. M., Lewis, C., Leake, B., Flaskerud, J., & Bennett, C. (1995). Barriers to condom use and needle cleaning among impoverished minority female injection drug users and partners of injection drug users. *Public Health Reports, 110,* 166–172.

Obbo, C. (1995). Gender, age and class: Discourses on HIV transmission and control in Uganda. In H. ten Brummelhuis & G. Herdt (Eds.), *Culture and sexual risk: Anthropological perspectives on AIDS* (pp. 79–95). Amsterdam: Gordon & Breach.

Odets, W. (1995, May). The fatal mistakes of AIDS education. *Harper's Magazine, 290,* 13–17.

Oliver, W. (1989). Sexual conquest and patterns of Black-on-Black violence: A structural-cultural perspective. *Violence and Victims, 4,* 257–273.

Overby, K. J., & Kegeles, S. M. (1994). The impact of AIDS on an urban population of high-risk female minority adolescents: Implications for intervention. *Journal of Adolescent Health, 15,* 216–227.

Payne, J. G., & Mercuri, K. A. (1993). Crisis in communication: Coverage of Magic Johnson's AIDS disclosure. In S. C. Ratzan (Ed.), *AIDS: Effective health communication for the 90s* (pp. 151–172). Washington, DC: Taylor & Francis.

Penner, L. A., & Fritzsche, B. A. (1993). Magic Johnson and reactions to people with AIDS: A natural experiment. *Journal of Applied Social Psychology, 23,* 1035–1050.

Perloff, R. M. (1991). Effects of an AIDS communication campaign. *Journalism Quarterly, 68,* 638–643.

Perloff, R. M. (1993). *The dynamics of persuasion.* Hillsdale, NJ: Lawrence Erlbaum Associates.

Perloff, R. M., & Pettey, G. (1991). Designing an AIDS information campaign to reach intravenous drug users and sex partners. *Public Health Reports, 106,* 460–463.

Peterson, J. L. (1997). AIDS-related risks and same-sex behaviors among African American men. In M. P. Levine, P. M. Nardi, & J. H. Gagnon (Eds.), *In changing times: Gay men and lesbians encounter HIV/AIDS* (pp. 283–301). Chicago: University of Chicago Press.

Petty, R. E., Gleicher, F., & Jarvis, W. B. G. (1993). Persuasion theory and AIDS prevention. In J. B. Pryor & G. D. Reeder (Eds.), *The social psychology of HIV infection* (pp. 155–182) Hillsdale, NJ: Lawrence Erlbaum Associates.

Pisalsarakit, P., & Tillinghast, D. Stover. (1999, August). *The HIV/AIDS epidemic in Thailand: From mass media campaigns to community interventions.* Paper presented at the annual convention of the Association for Education in Journalism and Mass Communication, New Orleans.

Prochaska, J. O., DiClemente, C. C., & Norcross, J. C. (1992). In search of how people change: Applications to addictive behaviors. *American Psychologist, 47,* 1102–1114.

Prochaska, J. O., Redding, C. A., Harlow, L. L., Rossi, J. S., & Velicer, W. F. (1994). The transtheoretical model of change and HIV prevention: A review. *Health Education Quarterly, 21,* 471–486.

Pryor, J. B., & Reeder, G. D. (1993). Collective and individual representations of HIV/AIDS stigma. In J. B. Pryor & G. D. Reeder (Eds.), *The social psychology of HIV infection* (pp. 263–286). Hillsdale, NJ: Lawrence Erlbaum Associates.

Pryor, J. B., Reeder, G. D., & Landau, S. (1999). A social-psychological analysis of HIV-related stigma: A two factor theory. *American Behavioral Scientist, 42,* 1193–1211.

Pryor, J. B., Reeder, G. D., Vinacco, R., Jr., & Kott, T. L. (1989). The instrumental and symbolic functions of attitudes toward persons with AIDS. *Journal of Applied Social Psychology, 19,* 377–404.

Ratzan, S. C., & Payne, J. G. (1993). Thinking globally, acting locally: AIDS Action 2000 Plan. In S. C. Ratzan (Ed.), *AIDS: Effective health communication for the 90s* (pp. 233–254). Washington, DC: Taylor & Francis.

Reel, B. W., & Thompson, T. L. (1994). A test of the effectiveness of strategies for talking about AIDS and condom use. *Journal of Applied Communication Research, 22,* 127–140.

Reichert, T., Lambiase, J., Morgan, S., Carstarphen, M., & Zavoina, S. (1999). Cheesecake and beefcake: No matter how you slice it, sexual explicitness in advertising continues to increase. *Journalism & Mass Communication Quarterly, 76,* 7–20.

Reinecke, J., Schmidt, P., & Ajzen, I. (1996). Application of the theory of planned behavior to adolescents' condom use: A panel study. *Journal of Applied Social Psychology, 26,* 749–772.

Reisen, C. A., & Poppen, P. J. (1995). College women and condom use: Importance of partner relationship. *Journal of Applied Social Psychology, 25,* 1485–1498.

Roberts, W. R. (Trans.). (1954). *Aristotle.* New York: Modern Library.

Rogers, E. M. (1995). *Diffusion of innovations* (4th ed.). New York: The Free Press.

Rogers, E. M., Dearing, J. W., Rao, N., Campo, S., Meyer, G., Betts, G. J. F., & Casey, M. K. (1995). Communication and community in a city under siege: The AIDS epidemic in San Francisco. *Communication Research, 22,* 664–678.

Rogers, E. M., & Shefner-Rogers, C. L. (1999). Diffusion of innovations and HIV/AIDS prevention research. In W. N. Elwood (Ed.), *Power in the blood: A handbook on AIDS, politics, and communication* (pp. 405–414). Mahwah, NJ: Lawrence Erlbaum Associates.

Rogers, R. W. (1975). A protection motivation theory of fear appeals and attitude change. *Journal of Psychology, 91,* 93–114.

Rogers, T. F., Singer, E., & Imperio, J. (1993). AIDS—An update. *Public Opinion Quarterly, 57,* 92–114.

Romer, D., & Hornik, R. C. (1992). Using mass media for prevention of HIV infection among adolescents. In R. J. DiClemente (Ed.), *Adolescents and AIDS: A generation in jeopardy* (pp. 137–158). Thousand Oaks, CA: Sage.

Root-Bernstein, R. S. (1993). *Rethinking AIDS: The tragic cost of premature consensus.* New York: The Free Press.

Rosenstock, I. M., Strecher, V. J., & Becker, M. H. (1994). The health belief model and HIV risk behavior change. In J. DiClemente & J. L. Peterson (Eds.), *Preventing AIDS: Theories and methods of behavioral interventions* (pp. 5–24). New York: Plenum.

Rotello, G. (1997). *Sexual ecology: AIDS and the destiny of gay men.* New York: Dutton.

Rotheram-Borus, M. J., Gwadz, M., Fernandez, M. I., & Srinivasan, S. (1998). Timing of HIV interventions on reductions in sexual risk among adolescents. *American Journal of Community Psychology, 26,* 73–96.

Rothman, A. J., Kelly, K. M., Weinstein, N. D., & O'Leary, A. (1999). Increasing the salience of risky sexual behavior: Promoting interest in HIV-antibody testing among heterosexually active young adults. *Journal of Applied Social Psychology, 29,* 531–551.

Rozin, P., Markwith, M., & Nemeroff, C. (1992). Magical contagion beliefs and fear of AIDS. *Journal of Applied Social Psychology, 22,* 1081–1092.

Ruggles, S. (1994). The origins of African-American family structure. *American Sociological Review, 59,* 136–151.

Rushing, W. A. (1995). *The AIDS epidemic: Social dimensions of an infectious disease.* Boulder, CO: Westview.

Sacks, P. (1996). *Generation X goes to college.* Chicago: Open Court Press.

Salmon, C. T. (1992). Bridging theory "of" and theory "for" communication campaigns: An essay on ideology and public policy. In S. A. Deetz (Ed.), *Communication yearbook 15* (pp. 346–358). Thousand Oaks, CA: Sage.

Sanderson, C. A., & Jemmott, J. B., III. (1996). Moderation and mediation of HIV-prevention interventions: Relationship status, intentions, and condom use among college students. *Journal of Applied Social Psychology, 26,* 2076–2099.

Seal, D. W., & Agostinelli, G. (1996). College students' perceptions of the prevalence of risky sexual behaviour. *AIDS Care, 8,* 453–466.

Seal, D. W., & Ehrhardt, A. A. (1999). Heterosexual men's attitudes toward the female condom. *AIDS Education and Prevention, 11,* 93–106.

Seibold, D. R., Cantrill, J. G., & Meyers, R. A. (1994). Communication and interpersonal influence. In M. L. Knapp & G. R. Miller (Eds.), *Handbook of interpersonal communication* (2nd ed., pp. 542–588). Thousand Oaks, CA: Sage.

Seibt, A. C., Ross, M. W., Freeman, A., Krepcho, M., Hedrich, A., McAlister. A., & Ferna'ndez-Esquer, M. E. (1995). Relationship between safe sex and acculturation into the gay subculture. *AIDS Care, 7* (Supplement 1), S85–S88.

Sellers, D. E., McGraw, S. A., & McKinlay, J. B. (1994). Does the promotion and distribution of condoms increase teen sexual activity? Evidence from an HIV prevention program for Latino youth. *American Journal of Public Health, 84,* 1952–1959.

Sepulveda, J., Fineberg, H., & Mann, J. (1992). Introduction. In J. Sepulveda, H. Fineberg, & J. Mann (Eds.), *AIDS prevention through education: A world view* (pp. 17–19). New York: Oxford University Press.

Sheer, V. C. (1995). Sensation seeking predispositions and susceptibility to a sexual partner's appeals for condom use. *Journal of Applied Communication Research, 23,* 212–229.

Sheeran, P., Abraham, C., & Orbell., S. (1999). Psychosocial correlates of heterosexual condom use: A meta-analysis. *Psychological Bulletin, 125,* 90–132.

Siegel, K., Raveis, V. H., & Gorey, E. (1998). Barriers and pathways to testing among HIV-infected women. *AIDS Education and Prevention, 10,* 114–127.

Signorile, M. (1997). *Life outside: The Signorile report on gay men: Sex, drugs, muscles, and the passages of life.* New York: HarperCollins.

Sikkema, K. J., & Kelly, J. A. (1995). *Community intervention to reduce AIDS risk behavior: A prevention program for women living in housing developments.* Milwaukee, WI: Center for AIDS Intervention Research.

Sikkema, K. J., Koob, J. J., Cargill, V. C., Kelly, J. A., Desiderato, L. L. Roffman, R. A., Norman, A. D., Shabazz, M., Copeland, C., Winett, R. A., Steiner, S., & Lemke, A. L. (1995). Levels and predictors of HIV risk behavior among women in low-income public housing developments. *Public Health Reports, 110,* 707–713.

Singer, M., Flores, C., Davison, L., Burke, G., Castillo, Z., Scanlon, K., & Rivera, M. (1995). SIDA: The economic, social, and cultural context of AIDS among Latinos. *Medical Anthropology Quarterly, 4,* 72–114.

Siska, M., Jason, J., Murdoch, P., Yang, W. S., & Donovan, R. J. (1992). Recall of AIDS public service announcements and their impact on the ranking of AIDS as a national problem. *American Journal of Public Health, 82,* 1029–1032.

Slaff, J. I., & Brubaker, J. K. (1985). *The AIDS epidemic: How you can protect yourself and your family—Why you must.* New York: Warner Books.

Smith, K. W., McGraw, S. A., Costa, L. A., & McKinlay, J. B. (1996). A self-efficacy scale for HIV risk behaviors: Development and evaluation. *AIDS Education and Prevention, 8,* 97–105.

Snowbeck, C. (1999, June 1). Best defense: Condom manufacturers promote new designs to keep AIDS at bay. *Pittsburgh Post-Gazette,* pp. F1–2.

Snyder, L. B. (1991). The impact of the Surgeon General's *Understanding AIDS* pamphlet in Connecticut. *Health Communication, 3,* 37–57.

Snyder, M. (1987). *Public appearances/Private realities: The psychology of self-monitoring.* New York: W. H. Freeman.

Snyder, M., Omoto, A. M., & Crain, A. L. (1999). Punished for their good deeds: Stigmatization of AIDS volunteers. *American Behavioral Scientist, 42,* 1175–1192.

Snyder, M., & Swann, W. B., Jr. (1978). Hypothesis-testing processes in social interaction. *Journal of Personality and Social Psychology, 36,* 1202–1212.

Sobnosky, M. J., & Hauser, E. (1999). Initiating or avoiding activism: Red ribbons, pink triangles, and public argument about AIDS. In W. N. Elwood (Ed.), *Power in the blood: A handbook on AIDS, politics, and communication* (pp. 25–38). Mahwah, NJ: Lawrence Erlbaum Associates.

Sobo, E. J. (1995). *Choosing unsafe sex: AIDS-risk denial among disadvantaged women.* Philadelphia: University of Pennsylvania Press.

Sondheimer, D. L. (1992). HIV infection and disease among homeless adolescents. In R. J. DiClemente (Ed.), *Adolescents and AIDS: A generation in jeopardy* (pp. 71–85). Thousand Oaks, CA: Sage.

Steinfatt, T. M., & Mielke, J. (1999). Communicating danger: The politics of AIDS in the Mekong region. In W. N. Elwood (Ed.), *Power in the blood: A handbook on AIDS, politics, and communication* (pp. 385–402). Mahwah, NJ: Lawrence Erlbaum Associates.

Steinhauer, J. (1999, September 1). Young, nonwhite, female and complacent about AIDS. *The New York Times,* p. A14.

Sternberg, S. (1999a, May 24). The epicenter of AIDS: Time bomb ticks south of Sahara. *USA Today,* pp. 1D, 2D, 6D–8D.

Sternberg, S. (1999b, August 31). AIDS drugs have limits, experts say. *USA Today,* p. 1A.

Stevens, S. J., & Bogart, J. G. (1999). Reducing HIV risk behaviors of drug-involved women: Social, economic, medical, and legal constraints. In W. N. Elwood (Ed.), *Power in the blood: A handbook on AIDS, politics, and communication* (pp. 107–120). Mahwah, NJ: Lawrence Erlbaum Associates.

St. Lawrence, J. S., Eldridge, G. D., Reitman, D., Little, C. E., Shelby, M. C., & Brasfield, T. L. (1998). Factors influencing condom use among African American women: Implications for risk reduction interventions. *American Journal of Community Psychology, 26,* 7–28.

Stokes, J. P., & Peterson, J. L. (1998). Homophobia, self-esteem, and risk for HIV among African American men who have sex with men. *AIDS Education and Prevention, 10,* 278–292.

Stolberg, S. G. (1998a, March 9). U.S. awakes to epidemic of sexual diseases. *The New York Times,* pp. A1, A14.

Stolberg, S. G. (1998b, June 29). Eyes shut, Black America is being ravaged by AIDS. *The New York Times,* pp. A1, A12.

Stone, J., Aronson, E., Crain, A. L., Winslow, M. P., & Fried, C. B. (1994). Inducing hypocrisy as a means of encouraging young adults to use condoms. *Personality and Social Psychology Bulletin, 20,* 116–128.

Struckman-Johnson, D., & Struckman-Johnson, C. (1996). Can you say condom? It makes a difference in fear-arousing AIDS prevention public service announcements. *Journal of Applied Social Psychology, 26,* 1068–1083.

Sullivan, A. (1999, September 26). What's so bad about hate? *The New York Times Magazine,* pp. 50–57, 88, 104, 112–113.

Surgeon General. (1988). *Understanding AIDS: A message from the Surgeon General* (HHS Publication No. CDC HHS-88-8408). Rockville, MD: U.S. Department of Health and Human Services.

Svenkerud, P. J., & Singhal, A. (1998). Enhancing the effectiveness of HIV/AIDS prevention programs targeted to unique population groups in Thailand: Lessons learned from applying concepts of diffusion of innovation and social marketing. *Journal of Health Communication, 3,* 193–316.

Swarns, R. L. (1999, October 24). Writer helps Soweto strip the shame from AIDS. *The New York Times,* pp. 1, A12.

Thompson, S. C., Anderson, K., Freedman, D., & Swan, J. (1996). Illusions of safety in a risky world: A study of college students' condom use. *Journal of Applied Social Psychology, 26,* 189–210.

Thompson, S. C., Kent, D. R., Thomas, C. & Vrungos, S. (1999). Real and illusory control over exposure to HIV in college students and gay men. *Journal of Applied Social Psychology, 29,* 1128–1150.

Trad, P. V. (1994). A developmental model for risk avoidance in adolescents confronting AIDS. *AIDS Education and Prevention, 6,* 322–338.

Umeh, D. C. (1997). Introduction: Fact and fiction about HIV/AIDS. In D. C. Umeh (Ed.), *Confronting the AIDS epidemic: Cross-cultural perspectives on HIV/AIDS education* (pp. xv–xx). Trenton, NJ: Africa World Press.

Ungar, S. (1989). *Africa: The people and politics of an emerging continent* (Rev. ed.). New York: Simon & Schuster.

Wagner, G. J., Remien, R. H., & Carballo-Diéguez, A. (1998). "Extramarital" sex: Is there an increased risk for HIV transmission? A study of male couples of mixed HIV status. *AIDS Education and Prevention, 10,* 245–256.

Waldron, V. R. (1997). Toward a theory of interactive conversational planning. In J. O. Greene (Ed.), *Message production: Advances in communication theory* (pp. 195–220). Mahwah, NJ: Lawrence Erlbaum Associates.

Waldron, V. R., Caughlin, J., & Jackson, D. (1995). Talking specifics: Facilitating effects of planning on AIDS talk in peer dyads. *Health Communication, 7,* 249–266.

Walters, T. N., Walters, L. M., & Priest, S. H. (1999). What we say and how we say it: The influence of psychosocial characteristics and message content of HIV/AIDS public service announcements. In W. N. Elwood (Ed.), *Power in the blood: A handbook on AIDS, politics, and communication* (pp. 293–307). Mahwah, NJ: Lawrence Erlbaum Associates.

Weeks, M. R., Schensul, J. J., Williams, S. S., Singer, M., & Grier, M. (1995). AIDS prevention for African-American and Latina woman: Building culturally and gender-appropriate intervention. *AIDS Education and Prevention, 7,* 251–263.

Weinstein, N. D. (1980). Unrealistic optimism about future life events. *Journal of Personality and Social Psychology, 39,* 806–820.

Weinstein, N. D. (1993). Testing four competing theories of health-protective behavior. *Health Psychology, 12,* 324–333.

Weisse, C. S., Turbiasz, A. A., & Whitney, D. J. (1995). Behavioral training and AIDS risk reduction: Overcoming barriers to condom use. *AIDS Education and Prevention, 7,* 50–59.

Wermuth, L., Ham, J., & Robbins, R. L. (1992). Women don't wear condoms: AIDS risk among sexual partners of IV drug users. In J. Huber & B. E. Schneider (Eds.), *The social context of AIDS* (pp. 72–94). Thousand Oaks, CA: Sage.

Wheeless, L. R., Barraclough, R., & Stewart, R. (1983). Compliance-gaining and power in persuasion. In R. Bostrom (Ed.), *Communication yearbook 7* (pp. 105–145). Thousand Oaks, CA: Sage.

Whitmore, G. (1988). *Someone was here: Profiles in the AIDS epidemic.* New York: New American Library.

Wiebe, D. J., & Black, D. (1997). Illusional beliefs in the context of risky sexual behaviors. *Journal of Applied Social Psychology, 27,* 1727–1749.

Williams, S. S., Kimble, D. L., Covell, N. H., Weiss, L. H., Newton, K. J., Fisher, J. D., & Fisher, W. A. (1992). College students use implicit personality theory instead of safer sex. *Journal of Applied Social Psychology, 22,* 921–933.

Wilson, T. E., Jaccard, J. Endias, R., & Minkoff, H. (1993). Reducing the risk of HIV infection for women: An attitudinal analysis of condom-carrying behavior. *Journal of Applied Social Psychology, 23,* 1093–1110.

Winett, R. A., Altman, D. G., & King, A. C. (1990). Conceptual and strategic foundations for effective media campaigns for preventing the spread of HIV infection. *Evaluation and Program Planning, 13,* 91–104.

Wingood, G. M., & DiClemente, R. J. (1997). Prevention of human immunodeficiency virus infection among African-American women: Sex, gender and power and women's risk for HIV. In D. C. Umeh (Ed.), *Confronting the AIDS epidemic: Cross-cultural perspectives on HIV/AIDS education* (pp. 117–135). Trenton, NJ: Africa World Press.

Wingood, G. M., & DiClemente, R. J. (1998). Partner influences and gender-related factors associated with noncondom use among young adult African American women. *American Journal of Community Psychology, 26,* 29–51.

Wingood, G. M., Hunter-Gamble, D., & DiClemente, R. J. (1993). A pilot study of sexual communication and negotiation among young African American women: Implications for HIV prevention. *Journal of Black Psychology, 19,* 190–203.

Winslow, R. W., Franzini, L. R., & Hwang, J. (1992). Perceived peer norms, casual sex, and AIDS risk prevention. *Journal of Applied Social Psychology, 22,* 1809–1827.

Winter, L., & Goldy, A. S. (1993). Effects of prebehavioral cognitive work on adolescents' acceptance of condoms. *Health Psychology, 12,* 308–312.

Witte, K. (1992). Putting the fear back into fear appeals: The extended parallel process model. *Communication Monographs, 59,* 329–349.

Witte, K. (1997). Preventing teen pregnancy through persuasive communications: Realities, myths, and the hard-fact truths. *Journal of Community Health, 22,* 137–154.

Witte, K. (1998). Fear as motivator, fear as inhibitor: Using the extended parallel process model to explain fear appeal successes and failures. In P. A. Andersen & L. K. Guerrero (Eds.), *Handbook of communication and emotion: Research, theory, applications, and contexts* (pp. 423–450). San Diego, CA: Academic Press.

Witte, K., Cameron, K. A., Lapinski, M. K., & Nzyuko, S. (1998). A theoretically-based evaluation of HIV/AIDS prevention campaigns along the Trans-Africa Highway in Kenya. *Journal of Health Communication, 3,* 345–363.

Witte, K., Cameron, K. A., & Nzyuko, S. (1996). *HIV/AIDS along the Trans-Africa Highway in Kenya: Examining risk perceptions, recommended responses, and campaign materials* (Final report of focus groups conducted with commercial sex workers, truck drivers and their assistants, and young men aged 18–23, at Malaba, Mashinari, and Simba truck stops in Kenya). East Lansing: Michigan State University.

Worth, D. (1989). Sexual decision-making and AIDS: Why condom promotion among vulnerable women is likely to fail. *Studies in Family Planning, 20,* 297–307.

Wulfert, E., & Wan, C. K. (1995). Safer sex intentions and condom use viewed from a health belief, reasoned action, and social cognitive perspective. *Journal of Sex Research, 32,* 299–311.

Wulfert, E., Wan, C. K., & Backus, C. A. (1996). Gay men's safer sex behavior: An integration of three models. *Journal of Behavioral Medicine, 19,* 345–366.

Zagumny, M. J., & Brady, D. B. (1998). Development of the AIDS health belief scale (AHBS). *AIDS Education and Prevention, 10,* 173–179.

Ziv, L. (1998, February). "I gave him my love, he gave me HIV." *Cosmopolitan,* 240–243.

Author Index

A

Abel, G. G., 34
Abraham, C., 30
Adelman, M., 89, 91
Agostinelli, G., 26
Aiken, L. S., 43
Ajzen, I., 17–18, 33–34
Alstead, M., 108
Altman, D., 126
Altman, D. G., 105
Altman, L. K., 1, 28–29, 112–113, 121
Amaro, H., 34, 49, 54, 57–60
Ames, L. J., 47
Ashery, R. S., 117
Aspinwall, L. G., 23
Atchinson, A. B., 47
Auerbach, J. D., 1

B

Backus, C. A., 36
Bailey, W. A., 2
Bakker, A. B., 36
Bandura, A., 35–36, 48, 84, 86, 90, 93
Barraclough, R., 41
Barron, J., 2
Basen-Engquist, K., 36
Basil, M. D., 74
Bauman, L J., 28–29
Baxter, L. A., 38
Bayer, R., 11, 98, 102, 104–105
Beck, K. H., 36
Becker, M. H., 17, 23
Bell, R. A., 41
Belluck, P., 61
Berger, C. R., 41
Bettencourt, B. A., 40
Binson, D., 73

Bishop, G. D., 127, 130
Black, D., 78
Blair, C., 64
Blake, J., 127
Bloom, B R., 1
Bolton, R., 33
Bogart, J. G., 59
Bonaguro, E. W., 98, 101
Bowen, S. P., 37, 52
Brady, D. B., 22
Brafford, L. J., 36
Brasfield, T. L., 111
Brenders, D. A., 26, 77
Brien, T. M., 36
Britt, T. W., 127
Brown, L. K., 55–56, 85
Brown, W. J., 74
Brubaker, J. K., 3
Buunk, B. B., 36
Bushman, B. J., 34
Busselle, R. W., 99
Bryan, A. D., 23, 43

C

Cameron, K. A., 64–65
Cantrill, J. G., 42
Capitanio, J. P., 99, 128, 130
Carballo-Diéguez, A., 46
Carey, K. B., 87
Carey, M. P., 87
Carmel, S., 22
Carvajal, S. C., 36
Catania, J. A., 12, 69, 73, 88
Caughlin, J., 37
Chan, D. K-S., 20
Chay-Nemeth, C., 122
Cline, R. J. W., 37, 58
Coates, T. J., 33, 46, 69, 109, 112

Cochran, S. D., 41, 51–52, 56, 72
Coley, B., 72, 79
Collins, B. E., 24
Connors, M., 54–55, 57–58
Coons, H. L., 54
Corby, N. H., 34–35
Crandall, C. S., 127
Crawford, A. M., 125
Curtius, M., 113

D

Dahl, D. W., 103
Daley, S., 62, 65, 99, 130
Dalton, H. L., 52
Daum, M., 78
Davis, D., 51
Dearing, J. W., 96–98, 105
DeJong, W., 104
Devine, P. G., 132
De Bro, S. C., 40, 42
Delaporte, F., 52
Derrida, J., 100
Diáz, R. M., 53–54, 59, 85, 112–113
DiClemente, C. C., 69
DiClemente, R. J., 26, 52, 54–55, 58–59, 108
Dockrell, J. E., 34
Donovan, M. C., 52, 99
Dostoevsky, F., 47
Dolezal, C., 46
Domzal, T. J., 101–102
Duck, J. M., 79, 94

E

Edgar, T., 26, 39–42
Ehrhardt, A. A., 117
Ekstrand, M. L., 33, 109
El-Bassel, N., 116–117
Elkins, D. B., 122
Elwood, W. N., 39
Emenike, I., 108
Etzioni, A., 11, 104
Evans, R. I., 36

F

Farabee, D., 57
Farmer, P., 49
Fee, E., 124

Fineberg, H., 2
Fishbein, M., 17–18, 20–21, 100, 112, 118
Fisher, J. D., 26, 84, 93, 106–108
Fisher, W. A., 26, 84, 93, 106–108
Fitzpatrick, M. A., 39, 41–42
Flora, J. A., 90, 98, 102
Fong, G. T., 87
Fox, D. M., 124
Franzini, L. R., 108
Freeman, K. E., 37
Freimuth, V. S., 26, 40
Fritzsche, B. A., 72, 74
Fritz, M., 13, 27, 44
Fullilove, M. T., 52–53
Fullilove, R. E., 50, 52–53
Fumento, M., 78, 99

G

Galligan, R. F., 108
Garner, R. L., 36
Garrett, L., 26, 77
Gerrard M., 34
Gibbons, F. X., 34
Giles, H., 81
Gillespie, C. C., 24
Gleicher, F., 80
Glor, J., 127
Glunt, E. K., 126
Gold, R. S., 47
Goldy, S., 87
Goldenberg, J. M., v
Goldman, J. A., 36, 88
Goodgame, T., 127
Gordon, C. M., 87
Gorn, G. J., 103
Gorey, E., 55
Green, F., 3
Green, J., 32
Greenberg, B. S., 99
Greenberg, J., 34
Guenther-Grey, C., 118
Guinan, M., 118
Guttman, N., 100

H

Ham, J., 59
Hammer, J. C., 38
Hammond, S. L., 26, 40

Harlow, L. L., 36, 88
Hauser, E., 99–100
Hays, R. B., 46, 112
Heckman, T., 47
Helman, C. G., 50
Helweg-Larsen, M., 24
Herek, G. M., 97, 99, 125–126, 128, 130–131
Hingson, R. W., 23
Hoffman, V., 40
Hobfoll, S. E., 56
Hogg, M. A., 79
Hood, H. V., 111
Hope, B., 47
Hornik, R. C., 106, 108
Hunter-Gamble, D., 59
Hwang, J., 108

I

Imperio, J., 97

J

Jackson, D., 37
Jamner, M., 34
Jarvis, W. B. G., 80
Jemmott, J. B., 9, 61, 107, 116
Jemmott, L. S., 61, 116
Joffe, H., 34
Johnson, E. H., 51
Johnson, S. J., 37
Jones, J. M., 9
Jones, E. E., 125

K

Kalichman, S. C., 3–5, 10, 24, 33–34, 37–38, 46–47, 72–74, 79, 92
Kaplan, B. J., 26
Katz, D., 43
Kegeles, S. M., 41, 46, 56, 69, 112
Kellar-Guenther, Y., 43
Kelly, J. A., 5, 33, 47, 84, 86–90, 93, 109–112, 116
Kelman, H. C., 74
Kernan, J. B., 101–102
King, A. C., 105
Kinsella, J., 96
Kirsch, I., 36
Krauss, B. J., 121
Kreps, G. L., 98, 101

L

Lamptey, P., 121
Landau, S., 129
Leukefeld, C., 57
Leviton, L. C., 16–17
Lipsky, D., 107
Logan, T. K., 57

M

MacDonald, T. K., 87
Maibach, E. W., 90, 98–99, 100–101
Mann, J., 2
Manstead, A. S. R., 36
Marin, B. V., 36, 59
Markwith, M., 128
Mattson, M., 24
Mays, V. M., 41, 51–52, 54, 56, 72
McGraw, S. A., 10
McGuire, W. J., 70–71, 90, 94
McKenzie, N. J., 58
McKinlay, J. B., 10
McKirnan, D. J., 47
McKusick, L., 36
McLaurin, P., 82, 114–115
McNeil, D. G., 117
Mercuri, K. A., 73
Metts, S., 39, 41
Meyer, G., 97
Meyers, R. A., 42
Michal-Johnson, P., 37, 52
Mickler, S. E., 26
Middlestadt, S., 18, 105
Mielke, J., 121
Miller, L. C., 39–41
Miller, J. B., 59
Misovich, S. J., 108
Mitchell, J. L., 52
Morokoff, P. J., 54
Morris, K. A., 78
Morse, S. S., 1
Moskowitz, J. T., 73–74
Myrick, R., 114

N

Nathanson, N., 1
Needle, R. H., 118
Nemeroff, C., 128
Netter, T. W., 99

Norcross, J. C., 69
Nieves, E., 103–105, 112
Norman, D. A., 15
Nyamathi, A. M., 55, 57
Nyakabwa, K., 62
Nzyuko, S., 64

O

Obbo, C., 64
Odets, W., 10
Oliver, W., 51
Orbell, S., 30
Ostrow, D. G., 47
Overby, K. J., 41, 56

P

Payne, J. G., 73, 98, 108
Penner, L. A., 72, 74
Perloff, R. M., 11, 70, 72, 118
Peterson, J. L., 47, 114
Pettey, G., 118
Petty, R. E., 80
Pierson, R. M., 98
Pisalsarakit, P., 121–122
Poppen, P. J., 38
Priest, S. H., 106
Prochaska, J. O., 69
Pryor, J. B., 74, 128–129

R

Raveis, V. H., 55
Ratzan, S. C., 98, 108
Reeder, G. D., 74, 128–129
Reel, B. W., 89
Reichert, T., 99
Reinecke, J., 34–35
Reisen, C. A., 38
Remien, R. H., 46
Roberts, W. R., 70
Robbins, R. L., 59
Rogers, E. M., 24, 33, 95–97
Rogers, T. F., 97
Rogers, R. W., 75
Romer, D., 106, 108
Rompa, D., 33
Root-Bernstein, R. S., 3, 9, 28
Rose, D. T., 47
Rosenstock, I. M., 17, 23

Rotello, G., 7–8, 21, 28, 33, 99, 104, 113–114, 130
Rotheram-Borus, M. J., 107
Rothman, A. J., 107
Rozin, P., 128
Ruggles, S., 51
Rushing, W. A., 4, 28, 51–52, 62–65, 95, 126

S

Sacks, P., 100
Salmon, C. T., 100
Sanderson, C. A., 107
Schmidt, P., 34
Schooler, C., 98
Schwartz, G., 127
Seal, D. W., 26, 117
Seibold, D. R., 42
Seibt, A. C., 113
Sellers, D. E., 10
Sepulveda, J., 2
Shefner-Rogers, C. L., 97
Shayne, V. T., 26
Sheeran, P., 30, 85
Signorile, M., 46–47
Siegel, K., 28–29, 55, 60
Sikkema, K. J., 55, 116
Singer, E., 97
Singer, M., 54, 59
Singhal, A., 121
Siska, M., 106
Slaff, J. I., 3
Smith, K. W., 36
Smith, P. M., 81
Snowbeck, C., 87–88
Snyder, L. B., 106
Snyder, M., 40, 43, 126
Sobnosky, M. J., 99–100
Sobo, E. J., 51–52, 54, 56, 58–60, 65, 85, 117
Sondheimer, D. L., 109
Spitzberg, B. H., 39, 41
St. Lawrence, J. S., 56, 111
Steinfatt, T. M., 121
Steinhauer, J., 2
Sternberg, S., 1, 29, 63, 113
Stevens, S. J., 59
Stewart, R., 41
Stokes, J. P., 47
Stolberg, S. G., 28, 50–51
Stone, J., 82–83
Strecher, V. J., 23

Struckman-Johnson, C., 107
Struckman-Johnson, D., 107
Sullivan, A., 131–132
Svenkerud, P. J., 121
Swann, W. B., 40, 78
Swarns, R. L., 131

T

Terry, D. J., 79, 108
Thompson, S. C., 26, 28, 79
Thompson, T. L., 89
Tillinghast, D. S., 121–122
Trad, P. V., 109
Turbiasz, A. A., 107

U

Umeh, D. C., 8
Ungar, S., 63

W

Waldron, V. R., 37, 41, 89
Wagner, G. J., 46
Walters, L. M., 106
Walters, T. N., 106
Wan, C. K., 24, 36
Weeks, M. R., 52, 59

Weinberg, C. B., 103
Weinstein, N. D., 17, 24–25
Weir, S., 121
Weisse, C. S., 107
Wermuth, L., 59
West, S. G., 43
Wheeless, L. R., 41
Whitmore, G., 1
Whitney, D. J., 107
Wiebe, D. J., 78
Williams, M. L., 39
Williams, S. S., 16, 40
Wilmot, W. W., 38
Wilson, T. E., 60, 80
Wingood, G. M., 52, 54–55, 58–59
Winett, R. A., 105–106
Winslow, R. W., 108
Winsten, J. A., 104
Winter, L., 87
Witte, K., 64–65, 75–77, 92, 107
Wolitski, R. J., 34
Worth, D., 58–60
Wulfert, E., 24, 36

Z

Zagumny, M. J., 22
Zanna, M. P., 87
Ziv, L., 24

Subject Index

A

Acquired Immune Deficiency Syndrome,
   see AIDS
Adolescents, *see* Teenagers
Africa
   HIV/AIDS and, 1, 61–65, 122, 131
African Americans and AIDS, 50–61
   persuasive communications, 73, 82, 92,
     114–115
AIDS
   cognitive decision theories and, 16–31
   crisis in Africa, 61–65
   definition of, 3–4
   ethnicity and, 50–54
   facts about, 1–2, 5–6
   gender roles and, 54–66
   interpersonal communication and,
     36–43
   overview of, 1–9
   persuasion and, 68–93
   prevention campaigns and, 94–123
   risky behaviors and, 5–7
   transmission, prevention, and, 5–6
   social psychological aspects of, 33–36, 43,
     46–48
   stigma of, 62, 124–133
AIDS Risk Reduction Model, 69
America Responds to AIDS, 105–106, 123
Attitudes, *see also* Persuasion
   functions and unsafe sex, 43, 46–48
   toward AIDS-related behaviors, 17–24

B

Black Death, 1, 95
Blacks and AIDS, *see* African Americans and
   AIDS
Blood transfusions, 7–8

C

Campaigns and AIDS prevention, 94–123
   gay men and, 109–114
   heterosexual youth and, 106–109
   injecting drug users and, 118–121
   international, 121–122
   minorities, 114–115
   theories of, 95–105
   women, 115–117
Cognitive dissonance, 82–83, 93, 132
College students, 26, 31, 40–41, 107–108
Communication, *see* Interpersonal communication; Mass media; Diffusion of innovations theory
Compliance-gaining, 41–43, 88–89, 93
Condoms, *see also* Safer sex
   attitudes, behaviors, and, 20–21, 23–24, 26,
     32, 36
   communication about, 13, 37–43
   crisis in Africa and, 64–65
   female condom, 116–117
   HIV/AIDS and, 6, 9–10
   persuasion and, 68–93
   social marketing and, 103, 106–109
   symbolism of, 59–60, 103–104
   Thailand campaigns and, 121–122

D

Diffusion of innovations theory, 95–98, 117,
   123
   criticism of, 105
Drugs, *see* Injecting drug use

E

Elaboration Likelihood Model, 80–81, 93
Epidemics, 1–2, 95

F

Fear appeals, 75–79, 92–93, 102, 107
Female condom, 116–117
Functional theory applications, 43, 46–48, 60, 66, 117

G

Gay men
    mass media and, 96–97, 103
    risky behaviors and, 5, 6, 7, 9, 21, 28–29, 32–33, 45–48, 53–54
    safer sex persuasive campaigns and, 109–114
    stigma toward, 53–54, 128–130
    values, politics, and, 95, 99–100, 104–105
Gender, *see* Women and AIDS

H

Haitans, 8
Health belief model, 22–24, 30–31, 43, 56, 66, 75–76, 117
    limits of, 24, 30–31
Heterosexual sex
    crisis in Africa and, 61–65
    HIV/AIDS and, 2, 5, 7–9, 24–28
    media scare and, 77–78
    safer sex and, 13, 19–21, 27, 37–44
    safer sex campaigns and, 106–109
Hispanics, *see* Latinos
HIV, *see also* AIDS
    crisis in Africa, 61–65
    definition of, 3
    transmission of, 4–9
    worldwide, 1–2, 61–65, 121
Homosexuality, *see* Gay men
Human immunodeficiency virus, *see* HIV

I

Illusion of invulnerability, 24–29, 56–57, 78, 79, 108
Information-Motivation-Behavioral Skills (IMB) model, 84–85, 93, 106–107
Injecting drug use
    campaigns to influence, 118–121
    HIV/AIDS and, 5–9
    HIV infection worldwide and, 64, 121

gender, sex partners, and, 54–59
    needle exchange programs and, 52, 57, 99
    stigma and, 129–130
Internet, 103, 131
Interpersonal communication, 36–43, 59, 66–67, 88–90

J

Johnson, Magic, 4, 72–74, 81, 92, 96–97, 122

K

Knowledge of HIV, 5–6, 51, 55–56, 65–66, 84–85

L

Latinos and AIDS, 53–54, 59, 113

M

Mass media
    news of AIDS, 26, 77–78, 96–97
    social marketing, 104–108, 115, 118–122
Methodology, 12
Minorities, *see* African Americans; Latinos

P

Persuasion
    description of, 11–12
    humor and, 91–92, 108–109
    importance of, 2–3, 11
    message characteristics, 75–83, 92–93, 107–109
    reducing stigma through, 130–133
    skills approaches, 84–90, 93
    source factors in AIDS prevention, 70–74, 92
Plans, 41, 89–90
Postmodernism, 100–102, 107–108
Protease inhibitors, 29, 74, 113
Public health, 11, 104–105
Public opinion, 74, 126, 131

R

Racism, 52, 61

S

Safe sex, 9–10, 86, 108
Safer sex
    campaigns and, 94–123
    crisis in Africa and, 64–65
    cultural influences on, 49–67
    definition of, 10
    emotional aspects of, 32–33, 43, 46–48
    innovative aspects of, 95
    interpersonal communication and, 36–43
    measurement of, 12, 18–20, 22–23, 34, 36
    persuasion and, 11–12, 68–93
    philosophy of, 10–11
    social cognition and, 15–31, 33–36
    snapshots of, 13–14, 27, 44–46
    Thailand and, 121–122
Scripts, 39–41, 43, 66, 88
Self-efficacy, 35–36, 54, 61, 76, 86, 90, 93, 117, 122
Sex
    abstinence from, 10, 108
    increases in, 8–9
    psychology of, 34, 39–40, 46–48, 53–54, 59–60, 62–65
Sexually transmitted diseases, 7, 9, 26, 28
Social cognitive theory, 35–36, 48, 66, 76, 117
Social marketing
    explanation of, 98, 123
    use in safer sex campaigns, 98–105
    values and, 99–100, 104–105

Speech accommodation theory, 81–82, 93
Stigma and AIDS, 62, 65, 99, 124–133
    reducing through persuasion, 130–133

T

Teenagers, 10, 26, 31, 86–87, 90, 106–109
Television, 10, 99, 106
Thailand and HIV infection, 121–122
Theory, 15–16, 33, 100
Theory of planned behavior, 33–35, 48, 57, 66
Theory of reasoned action, 17–22, 30–31, 33, 66, 80, 93
    criticisms of, 30–31
Transtheoretical model of change, 69–70, 118

W

Women and AIDS, 54–67
    campaigns, 115–117
    crisis in Africa, 61–65
    criticisms of research, 61
    female condom, 116–117
    feminism and, 60
    gender roles, 57–61
    increases in AIDS cases, 54
    individual differences, 61
    injecting drug use, 57–59, 61, 118–119, 121
    persuasive communication, 72, 80